BEYOND THE BACK

The Chiropractic Alternative For Conditions Beyond Back Pain

9 Top Chiropractors Share How They Help Patients
Avoid Drugs and Surgery Naturally

Book and Cover design by Prominence Publishing. www.prominencepublishing.com

ISBN: 978-0-9737453-2-0

First Edition: November 2016

Table of Contents

INTRODUCTION

"Your body's ability to heal is greater

than anyone has permitted you to believe."

While most people think of Chiropractic care as a way to treat back pain, in fact Chiropractic can treat a wide variety of health issues using a natural, drug-free approach. Chiropractic is about so much more than back pain. In the chapters that follow, you will learn some of the many ways that chiropractors are helping their patients lead healthier, fuller lives.

As a society, we are constantly looking for 'quick fixes.' If we have a headache, we take a pill. If our knee hurts, we get surgery. If we're depressed and tired, we don't look for causes, we just medicate – usually without thinking about whether or not there is a natural alternative.

The reason we decided to seek out the brightest and best chiropractors for this book is because I, the publisher, have seen firsthand the incredible health results that chiropractic care can offer.

The body knows how to heal itself. If you cut your finger, do you wonder whether it will heal or not? No. We know that a small cut to our skin will heal all on its own. It is actually incredible when you think about it. Chiropractic care supports your body's innate ability to heal itself.

There have been hundreds, if not thousands, of studies that have demonstrated how Chiropractic care helps heal conditions from headaches, to asthma, colic, foot pain, shoulder pain, knee pain and much, much more.

The Journal of the American Medical Association recently suggested that a person suffering back pain seek out Chiropractic care before resorting to surgery. It is truly possible to heal your body naturally, without drugs or surgery.

I, myself, was under my chiroprator's care throughout all three of my pregnancies, and I went on to have all three of our children naturally, with no drugs or intervention whatsoever. I believe that having regular, gentle adjustments throughout my pregnancy contributed 100% to allowing me to give birth naturally.

When my husband suffered a concussion, he went to our chiropractor. When our teenage daughter started getting headaches, she went to the chiropractor. Our family has been treated for everything from asthma to bed wetting to neck pain to migraines and more.

As you can tell, I am passionate about natural health care. It saddens me to think how often people pop pills without even trying to look at the underlying cause of their pain or other health issue. Did you know that acetaminophen is the most common cause of liver injury in North America?

It is my sincere wish that you benefit from the valuable information offered throughout this book. Each of the co-authors was selected based on their experience, education and reputation. You will see how passionate they all are about Chiropractic and you will read actual examples of how Chiropractic has helped alleviate many different ailments and diseases.

To your health,
Suzanne Doyle-Ingram
Publisher, Prominence Publishing

HOW TO HAVE MORE ENERGY AND GET MORE OUT OF LIFE

By Dr. Steve Polenz

Tell me about your practice and what kinds of patients you help?

My practice provides comprehensive care for my patients' health complaints. After 20+ years in practice I realized that we often need several types of care to get us well because often our health issues have multiple causes: physical, emotional, and nutritional.

I use low force chiropractic with clinical nutrition to get at the physical, emotional, and nutritional needs so that you can feel better and get healthier at the same time.

I have a practice where people come to me for everything from headaches to digestion issues to low energy. You could say I have a general practice. If you are sick, maybe I can help.

The result I help my patients achieve is feeling better AND living a fuller life. Let's say you come to me for digestion issues and you have bouts of diarrhea where you have to stay home until it passes. I want you to have better digestion, get rid of your upset stomach AND be able to go out and be more active in your life now that you are not trapped at home!

I want my patients to feel better and be able to do, see, experience more in their life as a result of my caring for them. I want to add quality to people's lives.

What led you to this field?

There are two events in life that led me to become a chiropractor.

I was in grade school and loved to play sports which I excelled at. However, I developed lower back pain and right hip pain that worsened to the point that I could barely walk, was no longer able to run, and could not kick a soccer ball without severe pain. My mom suggested that I see a chiropractor and I got amazing results with pain relief. Because of that I was able to get back to running and playing sports.

What was the other event that led you to this field?

Well, I was about 25, it was in my early years as a chiropractor and I was doing everything I knew to do for my own health, but my health declined and I had daily headaches, brain fog, digestion issues, knee pain, and foot pain.

At the same time I was struggling in my practice with why I would adjust one person, and get a miracle, and I'd adjust the next person and get nothing, no improvement whatsoever.

As my health declined, I remember it vividly, I sat down on the couch one night, and the bottom of my feet hurt so bad that I was rubbing them, and it was like somebody just walked up and tapped me on the head. It was sudden awareness where I realized I was having all these health issues, my feet were hurting constantly, my knees ached, and my digestion was terrible.

I needed to take naps every day, but not your typical naps, I was almost going into comas where I would be out for three or four hours, and I'd get up, and I couldn't do a thing the rest of that day. I couldn't get my brain focused. I couldn't get moving. With brain fog, I couldn't track conversations longer than ten seconds. I am not exaggerating on this, imagine not being able to focus on a conversation for longer than ten seconds! It made life really difficult and frustrating.

I hadn't realized all of that was going on until that moment. I stopped, and I could finally see it. I realized that something was wrong, and I had to figure this out. That's what led me to the clinical nutrition.

So I was having my own health issues and I was frustrated with why one patient would respond well to an adjustment and another would not. I got excited with the miracles, but the patients that haunted me were the ones that weren't getting better, and I was always trying to figure out why.

Through the functional nutrition I realized a lot of the problems that I'm adjusting people for seem like chiropractic issues, but are actually coming from some nutritional imbalance in the body, whether that's a toxicity, or an organ system imbalance, which is then creating the pain they're having.

I discovered that many physical complaints, like back pain, can come from toxicity in our body or from an imbalance in our organ systems. I was adjusting my patients for pain, which was a symptom, not a root cause and when I missed the root cause, my patients would not get better.

This blew my mind and I realized that for us to be healthy we need a multipronged approach to healing.

I was my first guinea pig and put this realization to work by seeing if adding clinical nutrition to my own chiropractic care would restore my health and it did! After I got my health back I dove into learning functional nutrition because I believed it was a huge missing piece for my patients' health and well being. I turned my attention to a group of my patients who were not responding to chiropractic care. They agreed to try functional nutrition with me to see if this new tool would improve their health. And it was so cool, every one of them got better!

My passion is to use the tools I have to discover the underlying cause of my patients' health issues.

The care I offer my patients asks 'why?'

Why do you have your health issues, is it from a physical cause? Emotional cause? Nutritional? Or all of them?

Once we find the cause or causes we can give the right care at the right time to help them get well.

Discovering this has allowed me to help people who before were going from doctor to doctor and not finding answers. Now I am able to help and as a result I am often referred the toughest cases.

How did you treat yourself with clinical nutrition?

I love how everything comes together when we need it. I realized that I needed functional nutrition for myself so I started studying it, and I found a group that was teaching a technique, because I knew I needed some framework to put it in.

At my first course on functional nutrition I met a doctor who had just moved to Seattle, and was opening up her practice so I went to them as a patient. I figured a great way to learn would be to get myself under care, and see if it works.

It was a period of about nine months getting myself healthier, and learning. Once I was ready to start working, I addressed a group of my ardent patients who I was adjusting for the same problem over and over, and I said, "You know what, I wonder if this would help, would you mind doing this?" At that point I was still a rookie, but they love me, so they said sure. Every single one of them got better, and those aches and pains that they had, that we kept trying to adjust them for, all of those things got better.

I gave my patients the same care I received and we all got better by improving our diets and using a custom nutritional supplement program that is tailored for each individual person. None of us are exactly alike and functional nutrition done well creates a custom program for every person and it matches each patients' unique needs.

I had a custom program for me and that gave me quick relief of my health issues.

How can chiropractic care help people have more energy?

By taking all the built up stress of life off of you!

The way I see it is that we all are wearing a back pack that we have had since we were little kids. Often when we have a fall, a bump, a car accident, or physical stress, a rock drops into our back pack. When we have emotional stress, like a traumatic event such as job loss, fight with someone, divorce, all the emotional stress of our lives, a rock and sometimes a boulder can drop into our back pack. Over the years our back pack can get heavier and heavier as it fills up with our stress from life. Having to carry the weight of our lives, having to carry all of the built up stress can really drain your energy!

Chiropractic care – the way I practice it – looks for the built up stress and how to relieve that. I find the stress trapped in your body and release it with an adjustment. I get to look in your backpack and remove the rocks and boulders so that you no longer have to carry all the weight of life.

Removing all the built up stress helps you feel lighter, calmer, and gives you more energy.

How are your patients' health issues affecting their body?

This is a great question! I have been in practice over 20 years and I have seen how overall my patients are getting sicker and sicker. People used to come to me with one or two health complaints that were fairly straight forward to help. 20 years later people are coming to me with five, six, or more health complaints that are harder to help them get over. Obesity is going up, diabetes is going up and the number of us walking around each day with chronic health issues keeps going up and up.

So how are my patients' health issues affecting their bodies? Their health issues are wearing their bodies down faster than ever before. The health issues we are dealing with today are wearing our joints out faster and causing arthritis at earlier ages. I am seeing more kids with pre-diabetic issues.

I am seeing a trend where we are aging faster than our years. It is estimated that if we keep going the way we are, the generation coming up will have a shorter life span than their parents.

What kind of testing do you do?

I will have a new video on my website shortly showing this.

I use body response testing where we challenge the body then read the body's response. What I just said is huge for our health. There is this really cool feedback system built into our body and if you know how to use it, you can ask the body a question and get an answer.

This is commonly referred to as muscle testing. I use the muscle test along with a challenge to the body which reveals where to adjust to release the tension and helps us to also find what nutritionals a person might need to get well.

So, let's say I was testing you. I would scan your body and your organ systems. I would look to see what organ systems are weak for you. Let's say it's your liver, and then I would figure out why. Many of us might have some chemical toxicity or heavy metals, or we have some sort of imbalance in the immune system where there's an overgrowth of bacteria, or viruses, or parasites. With muscle testing I find the appropriate nutritional supplements to help balance that. In the treatment plan we couple the diet with very specifically and carefully selected supplements to rebuild a person.

In this process we're cleaning up those things that we call the stressors, like the chemicals, the metals, and the viruses because they are the energies that are weakening you and creating health problems. Then at the same time we're working to rebuild and repair you.

Can you tell me more about muscle testing?

The traditional way it's done is this: I'm standing in front of you, and you've got your arm stretched out at ninety degrees from your body. I press down on your arm, and you resist; we see if your muscle is strong or weak.

For example, let's say I touch over your liver area on your right lower ribs. If your liver is not at 100% when I touch the liver points, and then I press on your arm because your liver is weak it tells the body, "Hey, I am weak here," and the neurological reflex in your body shuts down the muscle, and then your arm goes weak, and you can't hold it up. My patients love this! They can see what areas of their body are strong and what is weak. And they can see us make a weak area strong. They see how they feel better in the following days, weeks, months as they regain their health.

It is a simple feedback from the body, but you can use questions. Literally, it's as simple as this. I'm checking a patient, and I'm asking is this a structural problem? Do I need to adjust for this, or is this a nutritional issue? Is this emotional? And I get a weak muscle test which means no, I get another no, then on the last question I get a strong muscle response which means yes. So, then I can know where to go, and what realm and what tools to use for a patient.

Wow. That is amazing. And it totally supports the theory that your body knows what's going on.

Yes. I describe it to my patients all the time, "This is how I get in conversation with your body." You know how you go to a doctor, and they listen to your symptoms, and they think they know what's going on, most patients at that point roll their eyes, because they're so frustrated with western medicine. So I tell them here is how I ask your body questions, so that I can use my educated mind, and my experience on what I think is going on, and then I'm going to couple that with what your body tells me it wants me to do.

What are some of the ways that you treat your patients naturally?

I always start with 'Why?'

When someone comes to see me I use muscle testing to see what is the 'why', the cause of their health complaint. Once I find that we then know what care to use to get them well. This is such a simple question and it directs care and saves someone from getting the wrong care at the wrong time and not getting good results. Unfortunately, I see this a lot, people getting the wrong care for their health problems.

I had a woman come as a chiropractic patient because she had neck pain. That makes sense: chiropractic care for neck pain. In her history she had seen 3 different chiropractors, a physical therapist, an MD and got only temporary results. When I tested her and asked her body whether the cause was physical, nutritional, emotional, her body said it was nutritional. I told her that the reason she had good physical care and was not getting better is because there was something else causing her neck pain.

We did a functional nutrition exam. We found a chemical toxicity/sensitivity was irritating her muscles. We developed a custom nutritional supplement protocol for her to decrease the toxins and take that stress off of her muscles. The result was that she got better and needed a few adjustments with all of her pain now being gone.

Had I adjusted her only, she would not have gotten better, I have seen this time and again in practice, the wrong care at the wrong time and the results are dismal.

1. I find the cause of their health problems: everyone is unique and needs customized care.

2. I find what care is needed to get them well and bring in other care as the body asks for it.

Can you tell me a story about a patient, before they came to you and after?

A person came to me with low energy and feeling constantly stressed.

I started by checking her for what care she needed and found that she needed adjusting for general tension in her body, and for emotional stress she was hanging on to. As I assessed her, I found where to adjust to release the general tension. Then, when we tested her for emotional stress we found that we needed to focus on certain times in her life. This is really cool because we usually do not have to know why and we do not have to talk about past painful events. We just need to focus on "when you were 13 years old" and whatever other age comes up. We adjust for what shows up at that age and often a patient will feel lighter and more relaxed.

This treatment has spanned over several months, and this patient now has more energy, feels less stressed, is able to work more hours, and is repairing relationships with her family that were battles before.

Earlier you described that you had a woman come in as a chiropractic patient because she had neck pain. In her history, she had seen three different chiropractors, a physical therapist, a medical doctor, and she only ever got temporary results. So, you tested her, and asked her body whether the cause was physical, nutritional, emotional, and her body said it was nutritional. So tell me about what happened next.

So, first off, that sets up a red flag for me. Anybody who's had that many different types of physical care for what seems to be a physical pain, and it hasn't gotten better, 99% of the time they miss the true cause of it.

So, I wasn't surprised when I saw it was a nutritional issue. I had to tell her, "Look, this is what I believe. You've gotten all this type of care, and you haven't gotten better. If I adjust you, you're not going to get better. You're going to spend time and money, and we're both going to be frustrated. I believe your pain is coming from a nutritional cause, so I recommend that we do a nutritional examination for you."

So in this case I was switching the patient from the mindset of assuming she needed chiropractic care, to being willing to follow a clinical nutrition care plan.

After discussing what I believed would be the benefits of clinical nutrition, I explained muscle testing to the patient, and we began the examination. In this case as soon as I touched her neck her arm went completely weak. To find out what was causing it, I put the supplements right next to her body, with her holding them, then I touched her neck, and I tested her muscle, and she was rock solid strong, she could turn and move her head, and she had less pain.

So with physical pain it's immediate. We get to see that change.

After she started her custom supplement protocol we had regular visits to monitor her progress. On follow up visits I watched to see that the supplements are working which means that she was responding well and her body was showing improvement. And I looked to see if new problems were coming up. This is like layers on an onion. You peel one layer away and there is another underneath.

By monitoring her on a regular basis we were able to change her program as her body needed it to keep her healing until her body said it was done.

This patient responded very well to the care. She hardly even gets adjusted anymore, and she holds her adjustments much longer than ever before. That is one way I know someone is healthier, they feel better and need less care!

Successes like this, where I can improve the quality of life for my patients, are exactly what I'm in business for.

You don't have to do any blood testing or anything to find out?

No. Blood testing reveals some things, but it doesn't reveal others. Blood testing is a powerful tool when used correctly.

With this type of testing, patients see very clearly that I can get them the answers, and I do, and they get better.

What is your best piece of advice to have more energy and get more out of life?

1. Eat organic vegetables and fruit – my patients who eat a lot of vegetables and fruit are happier and healthier – the results are right there.

2. Gratitude attitude – each day in a journal do the following things:

   • Write down 3 good/happy things that happened to you today.

- Write down how you made those things happen.

- Write down how you can repeat them.

There is too much negativity in our lives and not enough positivity. This exercise puts positive messages into your life.

When you write down 3 things that were good about your day you show yourself that no matter how bad your day may have been, there are positive things that happen to you each day - stop and notice them. Then, when you write down how you made those things happen for you, you realize that you played a role in making them happen, AND, that you can make it happen again, you can recreate it. You are a co-creator of your own life.

3. Get the free report I wrote just for readers of Beyond The Back, you can find the free report here:

   http://www.glchiro.com/beyond-the-back

In this free report I reveal:

- 5 hidden stressors that drain our energy AND cause most of our health problems.

- Why doctors struggle to solve our health problems.

- Simple natural care that fixes stubborn health issues.

- The power of **Functional Nutrition**

Go to this link for your free report: http://glchiro.com/beyond-the-back

Discover what is behind your low energy – this one report will surprise you and could change your health forever.

http://glchiro.com/beyond-the-back

I want everyone to know what is in the free report so that they can feel better now and protect their health for the rest of their lives.

Call me if you are struggling. Most of my patients come to me after having been through different types of care with little to no results. I love to find the cause of our health issues because that is where the answer to getting people well lies. Find the cause and use the right care and the chances to get better are fantastic.

About the Author

Dr. Steve Polenz

Green Lake Chiropractic and Nutritional Healing
9750 3rd Avenue NE, suite 103
Seattle, WA 98115
(206) 523-0121
info@glchiro.com
www.glchiro.com
Twitter: @GL Chiropractic
Youtube: Steve Polenz
Facebook: Green Lake Chiropractic and
Nutritional Healing

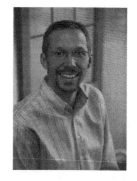

Dr. Steve Polenz, known to most as Dr. Steve, is a chiropractor, clinical nutritionist, and owner of Green Lake Chiropractic & Nutritional Healing.

Dr. Steve's desire to help and his drive to be an excellent doctor stems from twice having his own health struggles. His tenacity and love of learning spurs him to constantly improve his own skills as a doctor and to continually seek new ideas and healing approaches in order to help his patients enjoy great health.

After 24 years in practice Dr. Steve continues to share in his patients' joy as they feel better and get back to living full lives as a result of his care. He is joined by his wife and office manager, Theresa, whose compassion and dedication in helping people makes the office a wonderful place to be a patient.

Dr. Steve is also a mentor and teacher to his fellow doctors helping them get better results with their patients while having more fun at the same time.

You should know that Dr. Steve is 6' 6" tall and no, he was not good at basketball! Instead he fell in love with a short man's sport – cycling.

PREGNANCY

By Drs Matt and Jessica Thompson

Can you tell me a bit about your practice and what kind of patients you help?

Dr. Matt: Our practice is definitely a family-based practice, so it covers quite a range of ages and expertise, but we live in a young community, and so the large majority of our clients are roughly 40 and under, and lots of kids. That includes pregnant moms, and brand new babies, which are our favorite demographic. We certainly do have some people that are outside of that, but our passion, where we're at, where we live at, and just our expertise comes together to have that type of practice.

What lead each of you each to the field?

Dr. Jessica: Well, my story is that I grew up in it. I'm a third-generation Chiropractor! The story started with my great-uncle in our family. Actually, there are 39 Chiropractors in my extended family, and so it was something that I was introduced to from birth. Being adjusted right after I was born, and then growing up in the lifestyle of Chiropractic, getting adjusted on a regular basis, and having really good nutrition, and not being vaccinated, I experienced the benefits first hand. Also, spending time in my dad's Chiropractic office growing up, I got to see so many people see great benefits from Chiropractic care, and that just really fueled my passion to want to live that type of lifestyle, and also introduce others to it.

That's really interesting. Is it safe to adjust babies?

Dr. Jessica: I know that Dr. Matt will probably get into that a little bit more, but it's so important. When a doctor is helping a baby be born, the doctor is usually pulling on a baby's spine at around 60 to 90 pounds of pressure, and when those bones are so fragile and so little, it can cause the bones to move out of alignment, and cause pressure on the nerves, resulting in the baby's body not functioning as it should. The adjustments done on babies are very, very gentle, like the pressure you use to find out if a tomato is ripe.

Dr. Matt: Not only is the pressure of the adjustment even more gentle, but the adjustments themselves are very different. You can take any adjustment technique used on a newborn, infant or even pregnant woman, and use it on an adult, but you can't do the reverse. This is where seeking care from a pediatric, pregnancy and family Chiropractic specialist is important.

Dr. Matt, how did you come to be a Chiropractor?

Dr. Matt: A little bit differently than my wife. I also have a lot of Chiropractors in my family – there's around 20 - but I was not born into Chiropractic. My closest Chiropractor relative is my uncle. I saw his lifestyle, I saw how he made an impact in people's lives, and I really liked that. I liked learning how the body was self-healing and self-regulating, I enjoy helping others, and I have always been great with my hands.

There were a couple of different events that led me into Chiropractic, and took me to a better understanding of how Chiropractic can make an impact in people's lives. Like a lot of people, I had a sports injury in high school and I first sought care from the medical community, which ultimately missed a fracture in my low back. It was my subsequent Chiropractor that caught the fracture. It was a successful encounter, but it wasn't until I was in college that I truly committed to the profession.

When I was younger, I was diagnosed with ADHD, and I ended up being on medications for about 12 years of my young life. One day in particular I was in a hematology & urinalysis class looking at blood samples, and I saw strange crystals in my own blood sample. I thought this was curious so I brought the professor over and showed it to him. He looked up at me and immediately said, "That's medication built up in your system, what are you taking? What are you on?" My life was forever changed.

From that moment on I made a vow that I would never do that to myself again. It was such a scary moment for me, and seeing all of that in my blood told me that I needed to do things more naturally, healing from the inside-out. So I went to my Chiropractor and told her what was going on. She made a huge impact on my life, and here I am almost 15 years later. I owe a lot of the success I have to my paradigm shift that very day, but also to my understanding, and seeing that replayed for others throughout our practice. People can change their lives if they change their mindset and their paradigm.

Can you tell me a bit about how Chiropractic care can help pregnant women?

Dr. Matt: There's lots of different layers to this, and lots of different reasons why women would seek us out for Chiropractic care. A lot of times women come in because of obvious body changes; for example, they've got more weight on their joints because they're carrying two people. Their center of gravity changes, so it puts a lot of bio-mechanical stress on their joints. What we also know is that when the spine is misaligned, the hips are misaligned, and the sacrum is misaligned, and that creates a lot of stress and pressure in that area that does two damaging things to a mom:

Number one, it can pull the uterus out of its normal position which creates tension in that area. That makes it difficult for the baby to be in its most comfortable position not only during the pregnancy, but also during labor and birth which is very important.

Number two, the brain and body talk through the nervous system, which is held by the spine. We access the nervous system through the spine, so we know that when the brain and body are talking at a high level, free of interference, not only is mom's body functioning properly and doing all those things that it needs to do as it's growing and changing and supporting two lives, but also for the baby as well. So that's huge, and I think that once we do that, we set Mom up with an aligned spine, pelvis and sacrum. When she actually goes into labor, one of the biggest impacts Chiropractic has at that point is to allow that natural process to progress as it was meant to.

When the uterus is out of position, because it's attached to the sacrum which might be twisted, then you get into a situation where Mom does not progress during labor. We call that dystocia, and that's the leading cause for medical intervention for C-sections. To be able to adjust the spine and sacrum and just allow everything to be balanced where it should be and progress naturally is wonderful.

Dr. Jessica: Being eight months pregnant myself with my third child, I know that it's such a support to have Chiropractic care because the physical, emotional, and nutritional demands that are put on the body really affect moms. Getting adjusted can actually help the body deal with that stress at a higher level, and so I'm very thankful for Chiropractic in my life.

Do you do adjustments all the way up to the end of the pregnancy, or is there a time when you need to stop?

Dr. Matt: You can definitely do it all the way up to delivery, and right after. Now one thing that you do have to know is how to handle that, because you often need to do things slightly different. These slight changes have a significant positive impact in the outcomes. This is where it's important to have not only a Chiropractor who deals with kids, but someone who specializes in pregnancy, who has that understanding.

Chiropractic care helps pregnant moms so much, and the moms are loving us as they get towards the end of their pregnancy. They usually come in a couple of times a week because they're ready for their baby and they just want to have the best possible experience.

How does a woman's pregnancy affect her body?

Dr. Jessica: A few bio-mechanical things are: As the baby grows, it causes extra stress on the lower back (which we call the lumbar spine), hips and sacrum and it can extend that lower lumbar area, causing a lot of postural dysfunction and pain in that area.

Also, one of the things that happens is the mom's head comes forward, and so those are all things with the shifting and the changing of the body that can happen, but that can have an impact in how the mom is feeling and also how her body's functioning. Like Dr. Matt said, center of gravity can change, causing shifting of the entire spine. There is also a change in hormones, and one in particular called relaxin, that relaxes joints and ligaments. This increase in relaxin can cause joints to more easily move out of correct alignment, but is necessary as the body shifts, grows and changes to accommodate the growth of the baby.

It sounds like having adjustments during pregnancy, that might even help Mom after the baby is born, too.

Dr. Matt: Oh, definitely. It's all about doing things to prepare Mom for the birth. The whole process begins when she becomes pregnant, and all the way through post-partum. All the things that she can do to put herself in the best position to actually have the birth, are the same things that are going to help her heal even quicker. Chiropractic care addresses part of that, but she's also got to be moving and doing some other things, and we'll talk about that with our ten tips a little bit later.

Dr. Jessica: It's like the birth is a marathon, and getting prepared and ready for that. Chiropractic is part a big part of the training for that marathon.

What is a misconception that people have about natural childbirth?

Dr. Matt: I would say that probably the biggest misconception that I see is that women especially, and the families in general, think that they're unequipped, and that they're not capable of going through natural pregnancy and birth. I think that society has been conditioned to believe this. Obviously you might have circumstances that are out of your control that you need emergency care for, but that should count for a very small percentage of births. I think that women, and couples in general, just aren't empowered.

Dr. Jessica: Most often times when I tell people that I'm having a natural childbirth for the third time, they say, "Wow, how could you handle the pain of that?" or, "That seems like it would be so hard," and really my labors have been very easy, and I can attribute that to Chiropractic care. On that same point, it's that people think that natural childbirth is too hard or painful for them to endure.

Do your patients typically see midwives?

Dr. Matt: Yes, but we are a resource to the families that come in, so we have to meet them where they're at. A lot of them do use midwives, some at home, some in birthing centers, but sometimes people will come in and they don't have a midwife. We certainly educate our patients and are there for them as a resource so they can make empowered decisions.

What are some of the benefits of Chiropractic care during pregnancy?

Dr. Matt: Making sure that we keep the uterus level and balanced is very important, so we don't have any tension and pressure there. We also make sure the nervous system is functioning, free of interference, and that's probably the most significant thing, because when the nervous system is functioning at its maximum potential, then the body's going to be at its biggest potential, so Mom's sleeping better, she's recovering better, she's able to bounce back, she"s able to handle the stress and the discomfort, making it more comfortable for Mom.

Can Chiropractic care reduce the risk of complications during birth?

Dr. Jessica: Absolutely. When someone is getting regular Chiropractic care during their pregnancy, it's actually been shown to reduce labor times and it reduces the risks of C-sections. It also reduces birth trauma because when the baby is in the correct position to be born, there is not the use of forceps or vacuum extraction, or a lot of force that's needed by the doctor to assist that baby out.

Dr. Matt: I agree with that. We have lots of moms that have had kids prior to seeing us, and then kids while seeing us, and they all enthusiastically agree that regular care made a huge impact in their pregnancies and births. The number one reason that women have C-sections is failure to progress, called dystocia. There's a lot of things that fall under that category, and one of the biggest reasons that happens is because if the uterus is twisted and not in its proper position and allowed to expand, then the baby can't move and do all the natural twists and turns that it needs to do. Baby gets stuck, mommy's uncomfortable, the pelvis is in the way, the sacrum is in the way, whatever the case is, and then they say, "Hey, we need to go in, you're not progressing like you should, we need to start intervening." Intervening often means a C-section, and there's so many negative things about a C-section.

The C-section rate should be about four percent, and it varies around the country where it's at now, but it's significantly higher than that. Some hospitals are striving to be at or near 100%, which is absolutely horrendous.

In the United States, more babies die in their first day of life than all other industrialized country put together… by 50 percent, and that's a number that's scary and it's very, very telling. That's not okay with us, and part of our mission is to change that! I think that sometimes women are coming into birth and pregnancy unhealthy, but I also think that the medical profession intervenes too much. If we can treat birth like an event where we kind of stand back and watch and just do everything ahead of time to put Mom in the best position, then it becomes a natural process, just as God intended. This is in contrast to treating pregnancy and birth like a procedure, a medical diagnosis where mom comes in, she's pregnant and, "Oh my gosh, we can't get the baby out, we got to do this, let's start getting drugs involved, let's cut her open, let's pull the baby out." Some of the videos that I've seen, and some of the stories of families we care for would make your blood boil.

Ideally, we want the pregnancy and birth to be as natural as we can, and then veer off if and when we need to. When we have a vaginal birth, the head goes through the canal, it gets squeezed, all the bones that are in the head are meant to move, but when you squeeze the front part of the brain, the frontal cortex, it actually stimulates the brain in a way that progresses us and continues proper neurological development of the baby's brain.

Also when a baby comes out of the vaginal canal, that's when they're exposed to Mom's micro-biome, that's when they get all that good bacteria that they need to thrive. When we do a C-section, here you have this baby that is sterile, has nothing, has no bacteria, and then it's exposed to whatever's there. Whatever opportunistic, negative bacteria might be in a hospital. With a C-section, we are setting baby up not only to get sick, but also, long-term, if we don't start with that proper micro-biome, they can develop issues. If you're interested in learning more about this, there are all kinds of fantastic studies out there that have been published in the last five years.

When the baby's born, the new mom and baby should have skin-to-skin time, and it seems that we are getting away from these natural things, especially in the US, and it's so tragic.

What's the difference between the way an MD would treat someone compared to a Chiropractor?

Dr. Matt: Essentially it comes down to treating symptoms versus addressing the cause. Let's take Sciatic pain for example. A lot of times what MD's will do is just tell the pregnant mom that's the way it is. As another example, let's say mom is feeling nauseous and vomiting, so they give her some medications or some pills. That's about the extent of it. But if you get a hold of an MD who's progressive, they may say, "Hey, go seek out a Chiropractor who does pediatrics, maybe do some yoga," whatever the case is, but they're pretty limited in their scope.

Dr. Jessica: Ultimately, they're treating Mom like a bag of parts versus a whole. So if a mom is having carpal tunnel towards the end, we know that that head comes forward during pregnancy, which puts a lot of pressure on those nerves going into the hands and the wrists. If she is being adjusted by a Chiropractor, that carpal tunnel doesn't usually become a problem because we're consistently putting the spine in the correct position. An MD would just say, "Wear a brace at night time and we'll see how things go." So instead of looking at the whole picture, they're just looking at a section of it.

Dr. Matt: Yeah, they're more managing symptoms versus taking a look structurally at the cause, and at what can we do to increase Mom's function and her ability to have a healthy pregnancy and birth.

Dr. Jessica: Even with morning sickness, there's been so much research that points back to keeping the blood sugars constant, and also supplementing with magnesium, and a lot of medical doctors will just give them a prescription medication for their morning sickness, which is another toxin that can be transferred to the baby. Instead of going straight to medication we look at nutrition and other natural options.

Dr. Matt: Another thing that separates us – not every Chiropractor – but the way we practice, is we want to be a resource, and so we have a lot of resources in our offices. We have lactation specialists, we have midwives, we have resources to go above and beyond what our expertise is.

Dr. Jessica: We want our office be a support, and we're not going to judge if you decide to have a C-section. We want to support you in that process, but also give you information to make you think about things in a different light. So we're never in a condescending position, but more of an uplifting, empowering position.

Unfortunately, moms get so much unsolicited advice, so we just want to be a support to them and a safe place they can ask questions.

Can you give an example of someone that you've treated successfully?

Dr. Matt: We literally just this week found out about a patient who has been a patient of ours for years, and she's already given three amazing testimonies for our practice. She and her husband were trying to get pregnant, they were doing IVF treatments....

Dr. Jessica: And a lot of the difficulty they were having was because she had been on some very heavy fibromyalgia drugs and doctors told her that as a result it might be hard for her to get pregnant....

Dr. Matt: So she came to us because we specialize in pediatrics and we've been working with her to do things more naturally. She just came in this week and let us know that they're expecting naturally! It's such a joy to play even a small, humble part in that.

Dr. Jessica: This is probably a good point to talk about the Webster technique which is a technique that helps to balance and un-torque the uterus, allowing the baby to find and maintain their proper positioning in preparation for birth. We've had many, many moms go through that process in our office and be saved from having to go through a C-section because baby – with the help of Chiropractic – has now gotten into a more comfortable and natural position for birth.

Dr. Matt: As defined by the International Chiropractic Pediatric Association (ICPA), the leading pediatric and pregnancy authority, Webster technique is a specific Chiropractic analysis and diversified adjustment. The goal of the adjustment is to reduce the effects of sacral subluxation and sacroiliac joint dysfunction. In doing so, neuro-bio-mechanical function in the sacrum and pelvis is removed.

In other words, making sure the pelvis, the low back, and the sacrum are in a particular position so that the uterus is in its proper position, and it isn't torqued and twisted. When you have that torquing, the baby can't get in a proper position so it gets stuck somewhere where it shouldn't be, and the labor can't progress. Using the Webster technique, you take out the sacral subluxations, allow everything to be where it should be, and then the baby can naturally flip and turn and do whatever it needs to do to get prepared for delivery. It goes back to how to make an impact on reducing C-sections, reducing birth times, and intensity of labor.

I've heard about doctors pushing the baby into position, or trying to turn the baby through pushing the woman's stomach. That sounds really great that you're able to actually position the woman's body so that the baby can move into position on its own. That sounds safer and ideal, really.

Dr. Jessica: The Webster Technique is not painful at all. What is painful, though, is for a mom to go through that pushing and pulling of a medical doctor trying to move the position of the baby manually, and the baby's not going to want to move if there's not room in the pelvis for it to actually do that. So by taking a look at the uterus versus the baby's positioning, you can then make the uterus positioning ideal, so that the baby then goes, "Oh, well this makes sense, I'll go ahead now."

Dr. Matt: It gets back to the mechanistic versus the vitalistic view. The mechanistic view is little pieces. "Oh, baby's turned, I don't know why, let me just sit there and push on Mom's belly and see if I can force the baby to twist in there." Who is that comfortable for…? Nobody. Versus let's find out what the cause is, let's easily address and remove that, and then over the course of time, the baby will naturally do what it's supposed to do. It comes back to how would an MD treat something versus a Chiropractor, it goes back to the mechanistic view of health and wellness versus the holistic view. Everything's connected, and once we look at health through that lens, we'll be better able to serve the health of our patients and our community at large.

Dr. Jessica: There's one more scenario that came to mind as we were talking, and that is moms who have had multiple miscarriages. Oftentimes we will have moms come into our office after they've had multiple miscarriages and be really frustrated and scared about the whole process. By supporting that body in the parasympathetic – which basically runs our feeding and our breeding mechanisms in the body, and really focusing on the nerves that go to that uterus – we were actually able to help them have a successful pregnancy. So that's another thing that we've seen a lot of success with at in our office.

Dr. Matt: Let's talk a moment about the sympathetic nervous system (SNS) versus the parasympathetic nervous system (PNS). The SNS is the part of the nervous system that controls the fight-and-flight mechanisms of the body. On the short term, this is a great state to be in if there is imminent danger. Cortisol, a stress hormone, is released; pupils dilate; breathing increases, heart beat raises. If these physiological changes last longer than minutes, then our body becomes unbalanced and sick. The PNS is the rest-and-digest process of the body, also known as the healing state of the body. Think of it like this…The SNS is the parent who jumps in front of the family, ready to defend and protect the family. However, you don't want them to always be ready to fight. The PNS is like the parent who is there for long term health, ready to shape, mold and foster the health of the family. You need both, but they need to maintain a healthy balance

Most people in our society today are sympathetic-dominant, so they're going around stressed out. I think pregnant moms are even more stressed because not only do they have all the other normal stuff, they have prego-brain, and they have all the extra aches and pains and stresses that are going on in their body. Another way that specialized pregnancy Chiropractic care impacts moms is by tapping into that parasympathetic nervous system and balancing those two out. You don't want her to be too stressed out, but you don't want her to be too mellow, where all she wants to do is sleep. So it's finding that balance, and usually that means bringing them out of that sympathetic-dominant stress state, that fight-or-flight state. You can't stay in that forever, it'll kill you.

Dr. Jessica: Another patient that comes to mind would be a patient named Katie. She sought us out after her 37-week ultrasound where she found out that the baby was breech. She had already tried that external version where the doctor pulls on the baby and the mom's belly, trying to get the baby into the right position, and it was so painful for her, and it was unsuccessful. She came to see us black and blue from the procedure. She was frustrated because she wanted the experience of labor and birth to be a great thing, like she had with her previous son. So she actually went on a website called Spinning Babies, and she found out about the Webster technique, which Dr. Matt talked about.

When Katie first came into our office, she was very timid and a bit scared because she didn't know how Chiropractic could affect pregnant women, or even what the process was like. So through the course of the examination with her, and through that whole first couple of days with her, we were just really empowering her and educating her. After a series of adjustments, she would go and get checked out by her medical professionals.

After about two weeks of Webster adjustments, she was at 39 weeks, and found out her her baby had assumed a more natural position because the twisting and torquing of her uterus had been alleviated. Her medical professionals were unaware of the Webster technique, and they were really surprised that her baby had now gotten into the right position. She had a very fast labour, about three hours. So she had gone from facing a C-Section to seeking out an alternative method. Seeing success with that, she was just overwhelmed with excitement and so happy that she was able to have found us, and now is a vocal advocate of the Webster technique and of pregnancy and pediatric Chiropractic specialists.

Dr. Matt: Originally she had a C-section scheduled, and we were truly a last resort for her, and it went right up to the dot, the last doctor's appointment, where she had an ultrasound and the doctors were going to make that call for her, whether they were going to call off the C-section or not. She was able to call it off.

Katie writes a blog, she's called new patients for us, she's about to start a podcast, and she's going to have us on as guests. It changed her outlook on life, and she's definitely been huge in getting the word of Chiropractic and pregnancy out into the community and beyond.

Do patients typically come to you when they're already pregnant, or are they tending to be more patients that you're already seeing, or who regularly already see a Chiropractor who just continues to during pregnancy?

Dr. Matt: You know, that's a great question. I would say a lot of our patients are getting pregnant, and also a lot of pregnant women are seeking us out. Not only are we gaining a reputation in the area for being really good, but pregnancy & pediatric Chiropractic, as well as the Webster technique is on the radar now a lot more. We do have some patients that come from other Chiropractors to seek someone in particular, but that's a smaller portion that is growing.

What is your best piece of advice for pregnant women?

Dr. Matt: The best piece of advice I could give is to educate and empower yourself. That allows women, and their families, to think critically. Don't make decisions based upon fear.

What is your list of 10 tips for a healthy pregnancy?

1. Get checked and get adjusted on a regular basis by a pregnancy & pediatric Chiropractic specialist.

2. Exercise 30 minutes every day. That can come in many forms, it can be your walk, it can be stretching, it can be yoga, it can be anything, but just get moving, because we sit too much, we're too sedentary. Motion is the key to life, and we've got to get up and get moving. That's a great thing to get Dad involved with, too, and other kids if it's a big family.

3. Pay attention to your nutrition, in particular getting protein at every meal. I think that cravings might lead women away from protein, but protein is so important, it's the building blocks of life. Healthy fats are important too. We love grass fed beef, organic pasture raised chicken, organic avocados and organic, cold pressed coconut oil.

4. Increase your water intake. When there's more blood flowing, we need more water.

5. Get Dad or partner involved, because the more he knows, the more he's aware, the more he can be supportive of Mom, and it makes for such a beautiful process. One of the things that Dr. Jess and I did was to take a Bradley class together. We had already been through Chiropractic school, but Bradley is called Husband-Coached Birthing, and it's a great introduction, and it's like maybe a month and a half long, and we'd meet weekly, and it gets Mom and Dad prepared on what to expect, and educates them. Getting Dad involved is huge.

6. Question everything. Not in a negative way, but just ask why. So someone that says, "Hey, you need this, this, and this," ask why. "What happens if I don't do that, what happens if I do do that?" Understanding both sides of that.

7. Have a birth plan. In other words, what do you want to happen during the birth? If you're in a medical setting where you're vulnerable and

things are happening, you want to be in control. You want to know what's going on. If, for example, you don't want a particular type of intervention, having a birth plan can help you be articulate and strong in your preferences.

8. Develop a support system throughout the process. There's so many levels to this, not only are you tapping into family and friends, to help support you through that process, but there's a lot of people in the community that have been there and can help. This should include an advocate who is by your side during the birth, helping adhere to your plan while mom is vulnerable.

9. I think number nine would be taking time out every day – 15, 20 minutes, whatever that is—to destress. So that might be a yoga class, meditation, epsom salt bath, a good book, maybe going and getting tea with a girlfriend, whatever the case is, just taking some time away to just destress for a while.

10. Educate yourself. The more you seek out knowledge, the more certain and empowered you become, which leads to a healthier pregnancy and birth.

How can people learn about what you do?

We are in the process of developing a family based resource website at www.drsthompson.com. You can also email **drmattdc@gmail.com** or **jthompsondc@hotmail.com**. There are also some great resources at the ICPA. The ICPA is International Chiropractic Pediatric Association, and they're the leading, cutting-edge research-based group for pregnancy, pediatrics, and family care in the world. I'm getting my post-doctorate pregnancy and pediatric diplomate through them. Their website is www.icpa4kids.org

About the Authors

Drs Matt and Jessica Thompson

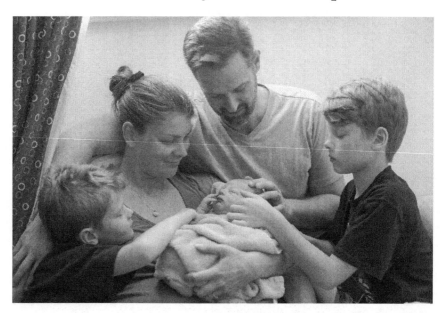

Dr. Matt & Dr. Jessica currently live in south metro Denver, Colorado with their three sons, the most recent coming at the end of summer 2016 with their third successful home-birth. They enjoy giving time and resources to their community, and do so in a number of ways. They are involved in their children's school since their first son was in kindergarten. They are also active members of their church, volunteering in the children's area, as greeters, with the Young Professionals and with the sports and recreation ministry. Drs. Matt & Jessica are also active members of the Highlands Ranch Chamber of Commerce. Currently, Dr. Matt is the chair of the Men of Business program, and sits as the newest member of the HRCC board of directors.

Drs. Matt & Jessica have always seen families in their offices, but are currently advancing their studies in pregnancy, postpartum and pediatric care at the post-doctorate level through the ICPA (icpa4kids.org) in an effort to better serve family, practice members, and the community at large. Both are certified in the Webster technique for pregnancy through the ICPA.

Although specializing in families, pediatric and pregnancy Chiropractic care, Dr. Matt & Dr. Jessica have tremendous experience and success with all things related to full expression of health and vitality. When the body is expressing health at 100%, not only do patients feel better, but most importantly, their body is functioning better!

RAISING SUPERKIDS

By Dr. Gil Desaulniers

Dr. Gil, can you tell me a bit about your practice and what kind of patients you help?

In our practice, we see people of all ages. However, our core focus and the majority of people who come to us are young families; almost 40% of our practice is made up of kids 10 and under. They're from all walks of life and come in for all different reasons, whether it's specific health conditions, health concerns, or just general wellness. Our main focus and our biggest commitment to them is to support their family's innate ability for optimal health and quality of life by offering them the best lifestyle education and chiropractic care possible.

What led you to this field?

I actually come from one of the world's largest chiropractic families: my extended family is 43 chiropractors strong and we've been in this profession for only 40 years. As you can imagine, growing up in that family meant you were adjusted starting at birth and under regular chiropractic care to maintain optimal health, so it was just normal. But as I grew up, I realized that it wasn't actually "normal."

When I moved away from my family and started experiencing the world outside of my family's chiropractic bubble, I realized how sick people were, how poor of a quality of life people were living, and the compromised lives people were living. When I woke up to that realization, I really saw and understood the necessity of chiropractic and the responsibility that I had.

There is a quote I heard years later that really rings true, and it brought me back to when I was 18 or 19 years old. My brother was starting his office as a chiropractor and I kept telling people that they needed to go see him, but I couldn't really explain it to them; I knew and understood that people needed to know what chiropractic had to provide, but I couldn't convey it. The quote is by the philosopher Voltaire and says, "The deepest, darkest places in hell are reserved for those who know and don't tell." It suggests a pretty heavy burden, but this quote reminded me of the great responsibility that I have. I didn't feel I could fulfill that responsibility based on where I was, but I saw the great need and necessity for it. It was at that time when I decided for myself that I needed to become a chiropractor to truly fulfill that responsibility.

I can't think of any better way to live my life and to earn a living than by helping others, and, as I said before, to support their family's innate ability to experience optimal health and live an optimal quality of life. I spend my life helping other people live the healthy life they're built for, they're designed for, and they're purposed for. This is why I embarked on my journey to go through university, Chiropractic College, and then onto my continued education with a focus on pediatrics and pregnancy. My focus on pediatrics and pregnancy allows me to start seeing them at the beginning of life, something that's vitally important because that's truly where it all begins and where you can have the biggest impact.

The motto in our office is "Start Healthy, Stay Healthy." We start chiropractic care as early as we can to start healthy, then understand and apply the tools and knowledge necessary to stay healthy for your entire lifetime, which is really the dream. Of course, it's also extremely important to me to help those who haven't been under chiropractic care all their life. For them, I hope to help start them down a new path of discovering optimal health and support them from that point forward on their journey to stay healthy for the rest of their life.

Is this a form of preventative care then?

I like to look at it more as optimal care. With prevention, you're still trying to shy away from a negative, rather than optimal care (or 'lifestyle care' as we call it in the office) where we are actually promoting a positive. Life is a continuum and we're always moving down this sliding scale toward optimal health or towards no health - death, essentially - so every decision we make takes us one step closer to being healthy or being sick. With preventative care, you're standing on that scale and looking toward the negative side, saying, "I need to know what can I do to not get over there." What this really ends up doing is just slowing you down from going there, but you're still going in that direction. On the opposite side of that is optimal care and optimal health: you're looking at the positive side and thinking, "What can I do to maximize my health? What can I do to maximize my life and optimize it rather than just doing the bare minimum in an attempt to prevent something?"

You have a workshop called "Raising SuperKids", what do you mean by SuperKids?

I actually open my workshop with a slide with big numbers that show 200%. This references a research study in which a particular intervention was shown to have a 200% increased immune system function over the control group, which is the average population, average healthy individuals. It ended up increasing to 400% better functioning in comparison to those people who were in critical care, have cancer and heart disease, etc.

We talk about it in the workshop, asking, "Who would like to have a 200% better functioning immune system?" Obviously, everybody raises their hands, but the catch is that you can't have 200% better function than what you should have. 200% better function sounds amazing - like the SuperKid I'm referencing - but in reality, that's just their optimal potential, whereas everybody else is not living to their fullest capabilities. That's where I was leading before when I was describing the difference between preventative versus optimal care. The idea of the SuperKid is that it's all about actually tapping into and releasing that super potential, going back to the beginning of our commitment to support the family's innate ability for optimal health.

Our bodies are designed to adapt to our circumstances to succeed and be healthy but because we live such a sick lifestyle, our "normal" is actually deficient. We don't realize it because we base our health on how we feel and base it strictly on symptoms, which isn't a true measurement of health. A fever doesn't feel good, but it's actually a positive thing. If you're constantly in fever, your body's always fighting something and always struggling to do so, so we need to look at why. A fever in and of itself is a positive thing, produced by the body to be able to fight infection. It's a great thing! It doesn't feel good, but I don't want to get rid of it because I want to make sure that it's a necessary function and supported in its fight so the body can heal as quickly as possible.

In short: SuperKid encapsulates when you're allowed the full potential to thrive. In this day and age, having full potential makes it seem like you're super human, you're a super kid, you have a super immune system, you're just amazing people. But for us, we call them Epic Chiro Kids.

Who is the workshop open to?

I host the workshop in a lot of different venues, from inside my office, to different professional settings, and free public workshops. I'm also developing it to have it as an online series!

Is it safe for children to be under chiropractic care?

It is very safe for children to be under chiropractic care. Really the only "negative effects", if you will, that have EVER been associated with chiropractic care in pediatrics is potentially muscle strain. And it's the same with adults when you look at the data and the research: if your body isn't aligned and functioning properly, there's going to be extra tension and by adjusting or working with certain areas, you're going to irritate those muscles just like you can irritate muscles by exercising...you can strain your muscles doing yoga. As far as research has shown, muscle strain is the only negative effect—the only other "side effect" of chiropractic care for kids is optimal health.

What sorts of things do you treat children for?

Well, the interesting thing is that I don't treat anything. I like to joke and say that I treat people with kindness, respect and authenticity - that's it. Kids will come in because of colic, torticollis, constipation, ear infections, autism, ADHD, anywhere on the sensory processing disorder spectrum, anxiety, allergies, scoliosis, etc... the list goes on and on. I make this clear to my clients and their parents from the very beginning: I don't treat any of these issues, but we see improved results for all of these issues. I look at what produces health in the body. Does a healthy body go to the bathroom? Yes. So let's make sure the body has everything the it needs for optimal function. If we create that, what happens to constipation? It doesn't occur.

We take that same approach with all conditions. We don't approach the condition itself, we approach the child that isn't living the life they're meant to. We structure our conversations with the parents around a salutogenic approach - an approach that focuses on factors that support health and well-being - rather than a pathogenic approach which focuses on the factors related to the disease, which is how our society treats conditions. What really creates health in an individual is how we focus which determines what care they need to achieve it.

How do you treat kids' health problems naturally?

I immediately think of this four year old boy that came in who was on a daily dose of laxatives. He had constipation issues since he was born and it got so bad that by the time he was two he was on daily laxatives. Obviously, the parents didn't want that as a long-term solution for him, but it was the only solution they had that was working. They had been to nutritionists, to naturopaths, changed a lot of his diet, been giving him probiotics - they've tried all these other alternative routes and all these wonderful things. When they first came to me, I told them to continue because they're still great for the body BUT since they weren't solving his problem, there was still a missing piece to the puzzle. To find it, we used technology in our office that measures nerve system function. By measuring his nerve system function, we saw that his autonomic system, which controls organ and glands, was stressed and dysfunctional. Through our course of chiropractic care, adjusting the spine allows the nerve system (which is protected by the spine) to reestablish normal connection and thus normal communication. Within two weeks, he was off his laxatives. Within two months, his digestive system had re-stabilized. I met his dad for the first time two months later and he thanked me for giving him his boy back. He said that when they would go on walks in the past, his son was sluggish and lacked energy, which was caused by the constant constipation. By allowing his system to function properly, he was finally able to have that energy and that happiness that a four year old boy should have.

I also cared for one little girl that had undergone 17 rounds of antibiotics for ear infections - ten within that last year - by the time she was five. Again, I don't treat ear infections, but we know there's a nerve that controls the opening and the closing of the Eustachian tube that exits from the top of the neck and in her case, that nerve was being seriously compromised. By correcting that imbalance and allowing the nerve system to reestablish normal connections with the opening and closing of the Eustachian tube, it was able to properly drain. Proper drainage = no ear infections. We don't treat the effect; we go to the cause of what is necessary for that body to function properly.

I take the same approach for dealing with kids with autism who were non-verbal and who've been able to start speaking. I have worked with a ten year old child who has numerous diagnosis, including a genetic disorder called DiGeorge's Syndrome. One of his complications is that he was supposed to be in diapers his entire life since he didn't have any bowel sensations. Within three months of care, he started to recognize that he had to go the bathroom and he was finally able to be potty trained. It sounds like a miracle but with SuperKids, it's really just releasing the actual potential that their bodies are designed for and allowing that nerve system to control and coordinate effectively.

How are their issues affecting their health?

I like that question because it cuts to the core of why we do what we do. It's not about the issues, it's not about the symptoms; it's about the effect on people's lives. For the constipated four year old, his issue stole his ability to express himself as an energetic, laughing, running, four-year-old, something that massively affected the family dynamics. It affects the families with autistic children even more and puts even more stress on them every day. Consider this: the average divorce rate across the board is 50%. For married couples who have a child with autism, the divorce rate in those families is 80%. When you can help these kids speak, calm down, and develop their motor skills, they can become more independent, calmer, and happier, and that changes the family's dynamic. It keeps these families together because they're no longer being torn apart by stress.

A lot of my main questioning when I meet someone for the first time revolves around this. Patient forms will get me the who, what, when, where, and why's of the condition, but what I really want to know is, "How is this impacting your life? When your body is functioning and you're developing this optimal health, what are you excited about? How is that going to change your life? What are you looking forward to being able to do again, do more of, do differently, or just do uncompromised?" That's the goal, to live that optimal life.

What's the main misconception that people have about chiropractic care for kids?

Unfortunately, there are many. A big misconception is that it is unsafe and unnecessary, which we spoke about earlier. Most kids don't have back pain or neck pain, so if we stick chiropractic in a box that says it's "only for back pain and neck pain and maybe headaches," adults even wonder why they would need chiropractic care. However, chiropractic care isn't about that at all. It's about the nerve system, and as we talked about, the spine is the protector and the conduit for the nerve system. We don't want to wait until issues develop, but if they do, we want to make sure that the foundation of function and thus health is functioning correctly. We need to think outside the box of health in general as well; I don't like to pigeonhole some of these conditions like autism, constipation, and ear infections, but when those things are going on we should make sure that the body's functioning correctly first so it can express better health.

Another misconception is that it's unsafe because their spines aren't developed and they're assuming that we adjust infants the same way we would adjust a 50 year old with advanced spinal degeneration that's trying to avoid surgery. We use completely different techniques and approaches with children: the techniques are extremely light and gentle. For example: when adjusting an infant, we use the tip of our pinky finger and apply the amount of pressure that you can put on your eyeball before it starts to be uncomfortable. Like I said, extremely light and gentle.

When should a child start chiropractic treatment?

Ideally, chiropractic care for a child should begin during pregnancy by adjusting the mother since her spinal and pelvic alignment and neurological health affects the baby's development, positioning and in-utero space. This all starts to affect the spine and the growth and development of the child depending on if there's something what we call in-utero constraint, which affects the positioning of the baby.

We want to start chiropractic care as soon as possible, so we can optimize development. It's never too early and it's always easier to start out on a healthier path when you begin early. As soon as a baby is born, their spine and nerve systems start to grow, develop, and adapt to the world around them. Just like you bring your child to the dentist as soon as they start growing teeth so you're able to address any potential problems early, you should bring your child to the chiropractor from day 1 so they can get checked and ensure they're starting healthy. And just like you bring your child to the dentist for routine appointments, your child should get checked on a regular basis to ensure that they are in fact staying healthy.

Do you have any other examples of kids that you've had success with that you'd like to share?

There is one that comes to mind. I often look at a poster I have in our office with an image of a mother pushing a stroller and carrying a baby. I had a client that said that she walked by one day and she saw that and said, "That's me." That very day, she was carrying her five month old through the park and he was just screaming his head off. For his first five months of his life, he screamed, non-stop, and she had no idea what to do. So she walked by the office, saw that picture, related to it, and then came in to see what kind of help we could provide. She had no idea about chiropractic care for kids even though she had been going to a chiropractor herself as an adult. I asked her why she didn't bring her child to the other chiropractor that she goes to, and she said, "I've been going there for years and I've never seen a single child in the office."

For the first month that she brought her child in, she would pretty much cry every time she left the office because she "...had a new baby and her baby was calm and happy." It's not a quick, one-time fix, but over a series of adjustments, those results of having that calm, happy baby lasted longer and longer until now he is a happy, healthy, active six-year-old boy, whom we still take care of in order to keep him healthy. His younger brother, who is three years younger than him, started care at four days old because the mother understood the difference and wanted him to start on the correct path from the beginning.

What is your best piece of advice for families looking for natural health solutions for their kids?

I have two pieces of advice, one being to simply get checked by a chiropractor. The second relates more to the way we look at health like I said before: taking a salutogenic versus pathogenic approach and actually understanding why something's going on and understanding why it's happening, like a fever. If you understand why the fever is happening and its benefits, we can understand that it's actually an okay, positive thing, not something that we need to get rid of or treat. For constipation, we want to understand why this issue would be happening by looking at all the components that are necessary for digestive systems to function, from the nutritional side to the neurological and control side of the body. In short, understanding what builds health in the body. If we can have a better understanding of why the body does what it does, then we can understand the intelligence of the body and support it in producing health. Not only will we achieve true natural health but we will build upon it exponentially to create amazing, epic, optimal health, rather than sticking in this pain-based cycle of treating symptoms after symptoms, a pattern that represses the body instead of building it up. It's a short-term versus long-term solution.

How can people learn more about what you do?

The best ways would be to connect with us on our website at www.optimumfamily.com or on our social media on Facebook, which is facebook.com/optimumfamily. Our Facebook provides constant information, success stories, knowledge, and answers to questions that people post on our page. They can ask us any and all questions that they want on those sites and we'll provide an answer.

About the Author
Dr Gil Desaulniers, DC

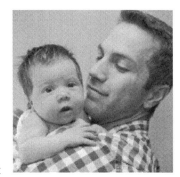

Dr Gil Desaulniers
Optimum Family Chiropractic
Port Moody, BC
778.355.3533
www.facebook.com/optimumfamily
www.optimumfamily.com
info@optimumfamily.com

Coming from one of the largest chiropractic families in the world (44 chiropractors in his extended family), Dr Gil has literally been deeply involved with chiropractic since birth. By the age of 9, he began assisting his father in their family office, helping patients and being witness to the changes and transformation that many people experienced in all aspects of their lives. This left a lasting impression that Dr Gil carries with him still today. Since making the decision to dedicate his life by helping people through the vehicle of chiropractic, Dr Gil has gone on a fantastic journey of learning, growth and camaraderie that brings him to the present moment. Along side his wife, Dr Marie, Dr Gil continues to learn and grow, but more importantly apply and teach the tools and gifts that he has been shown since birth. This unique life experience allows Dr Gil to have solid confidence and trust in the body's innate ability to heal. Approaching life and health from a vitalistic standpoint ensures that Dr Gil looks at the entire person when making lifestyle and care recommendations.

EPIGENETICS; A WORLD OF POSSIBILITIES

Dr. Stéphane Provencher

*"Tell your heart that the fear of suffering is worse than the suffering itself . . .
And that no heart has ever suffered when it goes in search of its dreams,
because every second of the search is a second's encounter with God and with
eternity."*

— The Alchemist

Tell me about your practice and what kinds of patients you help?

Within our Center we individualize the care for our customers. Our mission is to get to the root cause of the symptoms that they are bringing to our attention. Empowerment and education are the tools that we provide the customers to take back their health.

Gainesville Holistic Health Center (GHHC) provides a unique approach towards treating the whole person. Our whole "bodies" are actually made up of four distinct parts—physical, emotional, mental, and spiritual according to the old model. At GHHC we adopt a 5 distinct parts model according to the new quantum physic discovery. Dr. Amit Goswani PhD defined these new parts as Physical, Vital (or Emotional), Mental, SupraMental and Bliss (Spiritual). Each body should be balanced. This is the roadmap to health, wellness, and understanding our true being.

When our Physical Body is misaligned and/or stressed, the body ages more rapidly, breaks down more easily, and symptoms manifest known as "DIS-ease" of the body. Organ function is disrupted, there are issues with absorption and elimination for nutrients, and there is a feeling of heaviness, and stress on our skeletal frame. All of our reflexes - neuro-lymphatic, neurovascular to name a few - are compensating to give the physical body a chance to take care of the stressors. In other words, take the load off the skeletal part which needs to hold us and protect the nervous system.

The Vital or Emotional Body incorporates the nervous system, hormones, touch (and all other modalities), water and water release (tears), and water absorption (bloating or clutching from not letting go, feelings of lack, and trying to hold onto/control things too closely) when it is out of balance. This body can trigger illness based on holding onto unresolved emotional hurt.

A depletion of the Mental Body manifests as confusion, brain fog, ideas lost quickly, lethargy, lack of purpose, neuroses, doubt, a lack of work ethic, feelings of low esteem and low worth. Physically, it manifests as a lack of a menstrual period and little self-care. While an overabundance manifests as ego-centric, excessively driven, sociopathic, narcissistic, and having little or no empathy especially when it comes to work or success. This manifests physically in headaches and jaw aches.

When the SupraMental body is misaligned (which represent all the laws and archetypal context of physical, vital and mental bodies), all blueprints, beliefs, inter and intra personal rules and guidelines become faulty. We then operate our lives within an old concept of rules and regulations that was serving us at one time but is not now. I use this example in my center: If somebody ran after you to cause harm at the age of 2 years old, your set of defenses would be less than if you were

40 years old, right? The 40-year-old could run, kick, fight, call the cops, and use their body weight etc... but at the age of 2 you couldn't. If the SupraMental is not "updated" properly, you will react again and again with these now faulty beliefs or rules about danger.

When your Bliss (Spiritual) body is misaligned (also termed Wholeness by Dr. Amit Goswami), you may feel left out, or like you have not been seen or heard. There is also a tendency to put a high emphasis on how things look or how they appear instead of focusing on transparency and honest heart communication. There is also a heavy focus and over-reliance on doing, controlling, and the grasping of an exterior reference or relationship.

This model brings a multi-level of healing with a multi-level of evaluation and diagnosis to accomplish this whole-listic health. This is the reason why we chose to incorporate an integrative approach to address all levels of health within individuals.

We see everybody, at any age, from any type of boo-boo to serious illness diagnosed by medical/allopathic methods. Everybody fits into this Whole-Listic model and all can improve their health in all multi-levels according to the science of quantum physics. So we do not close our door to anyone who might suffer or wants to upgrade their status.

What led you to this field, Dr. Provencher?

I grew up in a family that held a somewhat medical mind-set. My father was a Chiropractor and my mother was an inhalotherapist; however, our lifestyle was more holistic. The nature vs nurture debate depicts my life. I was equipped with the genes, yet emotional and mental milestones altered their outlook; possibly a precursor to Epigenetics for me.

My earliest memories resounded with cries of discomfort and pain trying to establish my identity. As a child, I was subjected to constant bullying because of my issues with obesity. When my parents divorced, my reality was further altered and disparity occurred when I realized that my lifestyle would be changed.

This monumental event was one of the biggest stressors in my life that caused me to prematurely resign from my educational track and seek answers elsewhere. I took a sabbatical in Europe and came across the novel, The Alchemist.

This provided me with serenity and insight and made me recognize that my success was indeterminate and would only be constrained by my own limiting beliefs. I began to reflect on the age-old question of "Who am I?" and "What is my purpose in life?"

After I returned from Europe, I knew my calling in life was to be a healer, in particular, a holistic physician. A holistic physician that would incorporate various modalities of healing to find the root cause of the dis-ease. I recognized that the brain and of course the nervous system that attaches to our brain make up the most critical organ system in the human body.

The human nervous system is responsible for coordinating every movement or action your body takes. The nervous system is responsible for every function of the human body. In order for your heart to beat, your lungs to breathe, your food to digest and your feet to walk, your nervous system has to be functioning properly.

This awareness guided my studies and career in the field of Chiropractic. I was fascinated by the intertwined relationship of the body, mind and spiritual essence. I learned that 90% of all pain and dis-ease was impacted by emotions (unresolved emotional hurts) and it was not as much revelatory as confirmatory.

In particular, I was fascinated with the brain and its endless possibilities to govern all systems and organs in our body so I pursued a career in

Chiropractic Craniopathy. Do you have back pains, stomach pains, knee pains, etc? The problem may be all in your head... The skull houses 80% of the nervous system. There are 22 bones in the cranium interlinked via sutures. These bones have a required amount of movement within themselves as well as between each other. The movement is very small, but if this movement is dysfunctional, then it affects the conduction of the nervous system and the flow of the fluid that nourishes it.

These effects can be quite profound as the nervous system is the master commanding/communication system of the body. Nothing happens in your body without the nervous system's involvement.

I am an avid researcher; however, my passion for Epigenetics stemmed from our first pregnancy. In my humble experience, the creation of another human being is a divine gift that is bestowed upon parents. I took it as a serious responsibility to try to provide the ideal environment for my wife to nurture our children.

Like most parents, I wanted my child to come out healthy and equipped with idealistic genes. So I researched how to improve our child's blueprint, aka the "DNA." This drove my passion to research and learn from the experts within the field of epigenetics in order to help my own children and the children that I would be privileged to help in my center. Later, I found out that epigenetics can be influenced and changed not only via nutrition and chiropractic adjustment, but also by addressing all the 5 distinct parts of the whole-listic aspect of healing as mentioned above.

You also mention Epigenetics in your book, *Billionaire Parenting*. Can you explain what that is?

The beauty of being human is to go through the same patterns that others go through and have similar results, like having a baby. All humans go through the same physiological steps to deliver a baby but why do some have different hair color? Why do some have darker or lighter skin? Why do some hate the taste of kale or Brussel sprouts? Why do some become more introverted or extroverted than others?

The prefix epi- means 'above', so the science literally defines Epigenetics as 'control from above the genes'. The research community now understands and has shown that genes are incapable of activating their own expression and are not self-emergent or self-actualizing.

The different combinations of genes that are turned on or off are what make each one of us so unique. What turns them on/off is the source of epigenetics. In other words, they can be turned off (become dormant) or turned on (become active). It is the tools that the quantum doctors or holistic practitioners are tapping into to address health within oneself. Most importantly, these epigenetic changes can be inherited. Research has now proven that seven generations before you can influence the way your genes will react and turn on and off. Also, life circumstances/events and situations in life can cause and/or modify the genes to be silenced or expressed over time. So, environment, toxins, generational issues or challenges, even fears can be subcategorized under "stressors" which alter the expression of our DNA for generations to come.

Epigenetics, essentially, affects how genes are read by cells, and subsequently how they produce proteins, the building blocks of your physical body. With more than 20,000 genes, what could be the result of the different combinations of genes being turned on or off? The possible permutations are unimaginable! But if we could map every single cause and effect of the different combinations, and if we could reverse the gene's state to keep the good while eliminating the bad... then we could theoretically cure practically all dis-ease including cancer, slow the aging process, stop obesity, and so much more.

Here are some well-known examples of "stressors" influencing epigenetics:

1. **Contaminations, toxins, agents**

   a. Bisphenol A (BPA) is an additive in some plastics that is carcinogenic (cancer causing) and causes other diseases. Because of its effect on multiple dis-eases, it has already been removed from consumer products in many countries. BPA seems to exert its effects through a number of mechanisms, including epigenetic modification according to research scientists.

2. **Radiation exposure**

   a. X-ray, MRI, CT scan, SPECT

   b. Cellphone, computer, Wifi

3. **Diet, nutrition**

   a. Some studies done in Sweden and the Netherlands looked at ancestors who survived through periods of starvation and suggests that the epigenetic effect of famine was passed through at least three generations. These nutrient deprived populations are now diagnosed with diabetes and cardiovascular problems. A response that may have evolved to mitigate the effects of any future famines in the same geographic area.

4. **Pathogens**

   a. Bacteria, Fungus, Virus, Parasite, Prion

5. **Lifestyle**

   a. Smoking, alcohol, drugs

6. **Social environment (stress)**

   a. Childhood abuse and other forms of early trauma also seem to affect DNA methylation patterns. Some studies suggest that this may help to explain the poor health of many victims of such abuse that persists throughout adulthood.

7. Disease states

8. More

Some prominent researchers within the field of Epigenetics include Bruce Lipton PhD, Candace Perk PhD and Pamela Peeke, MD just to name a few. Candace Perk PhD discovered the molecule of emotion. She recognized that in order to create a thought or an emotion, your body needs specific nutrients to create neuro-peptides (molecules of emotion). A neuro-peptide is a neurological protein creating or producing a signal.

The interesting observation was that if you ate bad nutrients filled with chemicals or environmental toxins, the quality and specificity of that neuro-peptide will in turn trigger a bad thought and/or bad emotion within your body. The latest research also reveals that the bacteria in your gut will also secrete these same neuropeptides to mirror your thoughts. In turn, what you feel or think will produce a series of chemicals, hormones and neuropeptides in your body which the bacteria in your body can feed upon and amplify these frequencies to manifest the symptoms of dis-order or "dis-ease" in your body.

In Deepak Chopra MD's book "Super Genes," he reiterates this concept and explains that what you think and feel will influence your body's microbiome. Additionally, the nutrients you eat and absorb will have the same influence on your microbiome.

The microbiome in turn, has the capacity to influence your thoughts and feelings. It is a cyclical act. It will in turn trigger your genetic material to fold or unfold, creating a cascade of biochemical reactions which will produce either quality or sub-standardized proteins to support your body's overall health.

Pamela Peeke MD, described an experience on a "TedTalk" about a mutated mouse with two genetically alterations which created obesity and cardiovascular disease. The researcher fed some of these mice kale and other greens instead of the original mouse food. The results were astronomical. The offspring of these genetically engineered mice gave birth to mice without the predisposed genetic issues. In fact, these mice were non-obese and without cardiovascular disease nor did they show biomarkers for these diseases. As Hippocrates said, "Let food be thy medicine."

Your thoughts, your feelings, your food, the toxicity and your physical misalignment will alter the signal to the gene to express its self. These alterations will also be influenced by your microbiome and your blueprint/beliefs/rules and guidelines you built up since birth or even in-utero. These are cyclical until YOU break the patterns.

So, are you saying that it's possible to avoid getting sick even if your genetic makeup would indicate that you would likely get, for example, cancer?

The Human Genome Project began in the early 1990s and was initially focused on cataloging all the genes of the human body. The expected result was to correlate genetic variations with specific diseases in order to develop "gene therapy" which was supposed to be the future of medicine.

Billions of dollars were funneled into this project and the public was told this would single-handedly end heart disease, cancer, diabetes, autoimmune disease and hope seemed infinite. Scientists expected to find at least 120,000 genes with the assumption that there must be one gene for each individual protein in our body, in which we have at least 100,000 known proteins. On top of that, scientists assumed around 20,000 regulatory genes whose function was to "orchestrate" the complex protein assembly. When the Human Genome project was over, everyone was astonished by the fact that only 23,688 genes are responsible for the ever complex human body. So if we have 23,688 genes making 100,000 and more proteins, this means that one gene needs a separate signal to produce different proteins!

Research has now shifted into the study of epigenetics which focuses on how genes are expressed in our body and the causative factors.

Scientists like developmental cellular biologist Dr. Bruce H. Lipton have found that when the nucleus is taken out of the cell, the cell functions normally for over 2 months. It is thought in medical school that the nucleus harbors the genetic material of the cells and it cannot live without the "brain" of the cell. Well, Dr. Lipton showed that during that time, the cell is acting normally in its intelligent entity. This discovery leads to the conclusion that the nucleus is not the command center.

This analogy is common but illustrates perfectly the point: Think of the human life span as a very long movie. The cells would be the actors and actresses, essential units that make up the movie. DNA, in turn, would be the script — instructions for all the participants of the movie to perform their roles.

Subsequently, the DNA sequence would be the words on the script, and certain blocks of these words that instruct key actions or events to take place would be the genes. The concept of genetics would be like screenwriting. The concept of epigenetics, then, would be like directing. The script can be the same, but the director can choose to eliminate certain scenes or dialogue, altering the movie for better or worse.

So what contributes to the epigenetic signal, which in turn controls the genes? It is what you eat (real food or not), the environment of your living or work area, the person you interact with, your sleep habits, your exercise habits, etc. All these signals will influence your genes to turn on or off. Some will turn them on/off permanently and others just for a time and then revert back. Some research has demonstrated that bad epigenetic signals can influence cancer or Alzheimer's, which will be switched into the opposite state, away from the normal/healthy state.

An article by Dr. Mercola in 2010 suggested that, "according to Blair Justice, PhD, author of Who Gets Sick, genes account for only 35 percent of longevity while diet, exercise, stress and other environmental factors are the major reasons people live longer. Today, more than 95% of all chronic disease is caused by food choice, toxic food ingredients, nutritional deficiencies and lack of physical exercise."

How does Chiropractic care have an effect on genetics?

Your DNA is the internal blueprint which creates your physiology and in turn, creates the perfect healthy body. This process is where everything starts. Depending on the choices that you make and the lifestyle that you lead, you will greatly influence your status of well-being and health. As we mentioned above, your thoughts, feelings, food, environment, personal and inter-personal interaction, and radiation are simple examples of what can affect your DNA. Any or all deficiencies mentioned above will create a myriad of stress, interference and even blockages in the body's nerve system.

Dr. Issac in "Complementary of Biology" defines the minimum mass and energy that can metabolize and reproduce as a bion. Gaetan Chevalier, PhD renamed it a vion to avoid conflict with other researchers. A molding of the force of vions results in multivionic cells. This would allow for the development of large cells and even multicellular organisms. However, he states that this evolution is dependent on its quantic nature (e.g. nerve cells and brain cells). Proposing that the brain activity transferring to the nervous system to communicate its "will" has an impact on the minimum mass and energy that can metabolize and reproduce. In other words, if the nervous system's integrity, as a whole, is properly functional without interference or blockage, one would assume via this same quantic nature that the vion adaptation of function and specialization would operate within the field of health.

A study in 2010 published in the New England Journal of Medicine reported that our cells can interact the same way our nervous system does when it takes in sensory information and relays an appropriate motor output. Studies now show that our thoughts, stresses, social connections, diet, exercise, and exposure to microbes and environmental toxins all have major effects on how our genome is expressed. They now estimate this expression of genetics to be causing between 70 to 90 percent of all diseases.

Our digestive tract, respiratory tract and our skin (to name just a few places) hosts close to 100 trillion microorganisms. The amount of DNA from these pathogens or friendly bugs outnumbers ours by far. Some estimate the number by 100 times. Each DNA of the microbiome of our body will create a molecule or a signal that will impact our well-being.

Chiropractic adjustments (spinal, extremities, cranial, organ, reflexes and others) optimize the brain and nervous functions to each and every cell of the body. If the messages from the brain to the body via the nervous system are 100% functional, your body will, according to the above quantic nature, operate at its optimal level of health. Chiropractic care also optimizes the messages from each cell to the brain. The communication of our cells and nervous system to the expression of our innate intelligence is necessary within a clear and unobstructed path. This is why chiropractic care has such an impact on millions of lives and epigenetics.

Chiropractic not only improves the nervous system, but also the vascular, lymphatic, cerebrospinal, fascia, and muscular system. It will regulate or influence the limbic system (emotional center of the brain). The immune system is also regulated by increasing the amount of fighters against the microbiomes that may become out of balance, which in turn limits the bug's DNA to have an influence on our epigenetics.

Chiropractic physicians, in my humble opinion, have the most comprehensive study of the human dynamic and health available at this time under alternative healthcare. Chiropractic medicine understands the necessity of nutrition, motion, exercise, rehab, function, neurology and musculoskeletal and has specialization that goes beyond holistic and traditional care.

Chiropractic research proves the efficacy and the low cost of healing via a natural, drugless, painless methodology which accounts for the whole health of the person.

What is a misconception that people have about their health?

While we cannot define stress, all of our research confirms that the sense of being out of control is always distressful. As humans we have survived centuries due to our innate gift of being equipped with the fight and flight responses, aka "stress." These abilities are ingrained and are immediate reactions over which we have no control. They were originally designed to be beneficial to us by:

> ➢ Increasing the flow of blood to the brain to improve decision making; aka as hypertension, caused by our heart rate and blood pressure soaring.

> ➢ Blood sugar rises to furnish more fuel for energy as the result of the breakdown of glycogen, fat and protein stores; aka as diabetes.

> Blood is shunted away from the gut, where it is not immediately needed for the purpose of digestion, to the large muscles of the arms and legs to provide more strength in combat, or greater speed in getting away from potential peril or death; aka as obesity or ulcers.

> Clotting occurs more quickly to prevent blood loss from lacerations or internal hemorrhage; aka as stroke.

> Shallow breathing occurs in the lungs, which becomes symptomatic of asthma.

These examples are a myriad of immediate and automatic responses that have been exquisitely honed over the lengthy course of human evolution. These life saving measures facilitate primitive man's ability to deal with physical challenges.

However, the nature of stress for modern man is not an occasional confrontation with a dragon but rather a host of emotional and mental threats like getting stuck in traffic and fights with customers, co-workers, or family members, which often occur several times a day.

Unfortunately, our bodies still react with these same, archaic fight or flight responses that are now not only not useful but potentially damaging and deadly. Repeatedly invoked, it is easy to see how they can contribute to hypertension, strokes, heart attacks, diabetes, ulcers, neck or low back pain or worse, coping mechanisms such as smoking, drinking or other unhealthy distractors.

The body has an innate capacity to adapt and regulate itself to survive. The main direction or should I say, the main order of the brain is to survive. It will take all events/situations/persons, etc. into account and analyze it to which they are safe or a threat. Based on these 2 options, the brain will create a series of action/behaviors/changes in our physiology to put ourselves into a survival mechanism.

Dr. Hamer from Learning German New Medicine explored this phenomenon when his son died and he got testicular cancer. According to his research, he wasn't exposed or predisposed to have this cancer. Upon his thorough research, he found that our belief system and what we tell ourselves will manifest throughout our body. Louise Hay cured her cancer by doing affirmations. Dr. Joe Dispenza remodeled and healed several spinal vertebra fractures in 3 months after a Bronco hit him during a triathlon race.

I guess what people need to retain from this is that we have all have the opportunity to create "miracles" from our innate intelligence to heal ourselves. What you think will affect your health. What you feel will affect your health. What you eat or expose yourself to will affect your health. What you put on your body or smell or see or touch will affect your health. I guess the biggest miracle I see is the self-realization that my patient gets when they analyze their beliefs and come to the conclusion that they created this by themselves. The pain automatically disappears. When this self-realization occurs then we can work on the damaging factors and reversing them with chiropractic, nutrition, bioresonance and quantum physics, acupuncture, yoga therapy, herbology, Ayurveda, and more.

What is your best piece of advice for patients looking for natural health solutions?

All the great integrative systems of the body operate on a system of checks and balances. The autonomic nervous system has balancing antagonistic but complementary sympathetic and parasympathetic components. The endocrine system is regulated by feedback (positive or negative) making sure that if the thyroid is sending hormones, the adrenal glands are responding to the brain and letting it know that the signal was received.

Optimal health depends on good communication within the internal environment, as well as with the external environment. That holds true for all living systems, ranging upward from the atom to the cell to an organ to the brain, person, family, corporation, nation, and society.

No matter our daily tasks, these systems are in constant communication. If a problem occurs at one level, it can reverberate up and/or down the line. The key is to choose Whole-Listic and integrative health instead of the marketing terms of holistic, alternative, wellness, etc. Whole-Listic and Integrative healthcare utilizes the best therapeutic options from western medicine to complementary therapies and healing practices, such as chiropractic, herbal medicine, acupuncture, massage, biofeedback, bioresonance, biofrequencies, Ayurveda, yoga, meditation, PEMF and stress reduction techniques, to name a few. It offers a broad approach to healing that is patient-centered and focuses on the whole person: mind, body, and spirit.

Many complementary therapies and healing practices can help your overall health and wellbeing, in addition to helping you deal with your specific health issue.

For example, Yoga Therapy employs a multi-faceted bio/psycho/spiritual lens to identify possible causes of distress or malfunction and teaches self-directed tools to alter vital functions and promote a cascade of positive biological changes. The philosophy and practice is formed by ancient wisdom texts, scientific evidence and personal experience. Participants report experiencing global relaxation and re-connection with forgotten or lost parts of the self. Yoga Therapy designs customized preventative and remedial wellness programs targeting complex health issues such as grief, trauma, chronic pain, disability, disease and disbelief. It can also provide more general benefits, such as an internal sense of mastery and a more accepting, less reactive approach to life. Practicing yoga can lead to reflection and understanding of what guides our choices in life.

While you may be dealing with a specific health challenge, don't forget about your whole body, mind, and spirit, as well as your values and passions in life. Health challenges can impact our understanding and guide us to prioritize decisions in our lives.

Many people feel they cannot afford to pay for complementary and alternative medicine. However, if you look carefully you will see that insurance does not always provide coverage until your deductible has been met. Often people are responsible for a specified percentage of hospital stays. These can cost in the millions for intensive care or emergency visits! If you utilize your consumer purchasing power, you can determine if you would rather spend your hard earned money on one emergency visit or hospital stay or on preventive care which regulates the body's innate healing powers.

In the book, "Leaders and Legends of America," which I co-wrote with Louise Hay, Dr. Wayne Dyer, Dr. John Demartini, Bob Proctor, and Jack Canfield to name a few, I divulge the ultimate secret to optimum health: LOVE. Loving ourselves—love that is unconditional, non-judgmental, and open to new ways of walking through the world—enables us to experience love for others, affect healing, and watch as it heals the mosaic of the universe.

Healing occurs when we experience our connectedness to everything else, when we see the wholeness and perfection in all that exists. When we know such loving energy, our bodies, minds, and souls can experience true healing. For what is more deeply embedded, more powerful, and more impactful in human nature than love?

How can people learn more about what you do?

My dream is to create a multi-faceted model of health care under one roof for children. After many years of practice within the community, it dawned on me that in order to help families, the education and prevention must begin with the next generation and therefore I have chosen to shift my focus on children.

This mission is coming to fruition with the building of the Whole-Listic Children's Hospatal (Hospital + Spa + Gifted Academy) to address the primary stressors in a person's life and the societal issues that are currently facing the next generation. The goal is to have, under one roof, all modalities resolving health challenges in the Physical, Vital, Mental, SupraMental and Bliss body mentioned before.

The initial phase of the Hospital will focus on bringing in the next generation of children with its state of the art maternity ward. This will focus on the joys of mother-hood instead of the fears of pregnancy.

Additionally, the prematurity rates are on the rise, especially with the infertility rates increasing. Yet these populations have the least opportunity to receive alternative healthcare to address their weakened bodies. Our hospital will use innovative and integrative methods to help these most distressed babies thrive and regain their health.

Our facility will also incorporate innovative tools that help reduce stress for the children and their families. Children and adults alike who are obese or overweight are more likely to feel stress.

The obesity rate among U.S. adults in 2015 climbed to a new high of 28.0%, with another 35.6% of adults classified as overweight. This represents an increase of about 6.1 million U.S. adults who are obese. Children, regardless of weight or age, say they can tell that their parents are stressed when they argue and complain, which many children say makes them feel sad and worried. Parents, however, are not fully realizing the impact their own stress is having on their children.

Other signs of parental stress recognized by children are arguing with other people in the house, complaining or telling children about their problems and being too busy or not having enough time to spend with them. The primary manifestation of children's stress levels occurs when children have a difficult time falling asleep or staying asleep. Other physical symptoms of stress in children include: irritability, anger, lack of interest, motivation or energy, headaches, and feelings of depression or sadness. By 2025, Stephanie Seneff, PhD from MIT denotes that one in two children will be categorized with an autistic spectrum disorder.

It is also imperative that this Gifted Academy focuses on an under-served population. The stats regarding the post high school success of students with special needs is very poor. Currently, 80% to 90% of them are unemployed or underemployed. These are horrific numbers and our goal is to change them. The school will allot 35% of its enrollment to this under-served population.

The Gifted Academy will be designed to address the needs of the next generation of children. It will tap into their fullest potential by integrating the "whole-mind" and bring forth their natural talents in correlation with the type of learning style they thrive in (auditory, visual, tactile) in conjunction with individualized coaching.

The Gifted Academy will utilize coaching rather than teaching. Coaching is about the student. Coaching is unlocking a person's potential to maximize their own performance and bring out their true talents, "GIFTS".

Currently, in Los Angeles, STEM3 Academy took an out-of-the-box approach for a specific reason: All of its students have a learning challenge, like autism-spectrum disorder, Asperger's and ADHD. The students are especially gifted in subjects like math and science and have tested in 99% in the PSATS, but have fallen behind in their social and communication skills. However, the school chose to focus on their strengths instead of their "DIS-abilities."

This is a community effort; we would like to bring back the concept of "It takes a village to raise a child." This will be a community effort, a hospital for the people, designed by the people. We are asking for both monetary and non-monetary support. Our mission is to empower YOU with knowledge to take back your health. But you play the most integral role in the team. For further information on how you can help make this village a reality, please visit:

www.all4ourkids.org

www.billionaireparenting.com

and www.ghhcenter.com.

About the Author

Dr Stéphane Provencher

D.C., D.I.C.S., C.K.T.P.
Author, Speaker, Researcher, Instructor, and
Whole-Listic Physician
www.billionaireparenting.com
www.all4ourkids.org
www.drstephane.com
www.ghhcenter.com
Social Media:
http://www.linkedin.com/in/drstephane
https://www.facebook.com/drstephane
https://www.facebook.com/ghhctr

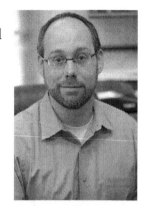

For many years, Stéphane Provencher's earliest memories resounded with cries of pain and discomfort. Massively obese and bullied throughout childhood, he knew only one thing for certain: He was not normal. "By the time my parents divorced, it was clear that any personal roadmap I might have developed had been shattered, my apparent destiny no more than a vague memory wrapped in the solitude of despair. It was not until years later, after leaving school and traveling through Europe, that I read *The Alchemist* and discovered that my limiting beliefs were no more than illusion and began to ask *Who am I? Why am I here?*

Now able to see his past cast in the colors of a rainbow rather than the prior swathe of black, Stéphane recalled how his gift for intuiting where people held pain had enabled him to look deep inside their souls, feel their feelings, and help them heal their wounds. This awareness guided him in his dedicated studies and career in chiropractic, through which he began to truly understand the intertwined relationship among the body, mind, and spirit. For Stéphane, learning that emotions—not physical ailments—actually cause 90% of all pain, all dis-ease, was not as much revelatory as confirmatory.

It was the staggering realization that emitting or sending frequencies of love can restore proper balance, however, that forever changed Stéphane Provencher's life and the lives of those he serves. "I am 100% clear that I am only a vehicle. My commitment and passion is to guide as many as possible to wellness through self-love and knowledge, and I invite all of you to join me on this extraordinary journey of the soul."

Dr. Stéphane is featured among Wayne Dyer, Louise Hay, Tony Robbing, Bill Gates, Maya Angelou, Brian Tracy, Tom Hopkins, Bob Proctor, Jack Nicklaus and many other in the **Leaders & Legends – One life, success, health, wealth and happiness** book from the America's Legacy Library released September 2015.

From a young age, Dr. Stéphane's dream was to unite a multi-faceted model of health care in one place. Dr. Stéphane is the vice-president of the **Whole-Listic Children's Foundation** and wrote a book called Billionaire Parenting – Give your Kids the World in 2014 (**www.billionaireparenting.com**). With the building of the Whole-Listic Children's Hospital underway, this dream is now coming to fruition.

HEALING KNEES NATURALLY

By Dr. David Sundy

Dr. Sundy, you have a very interesting specialty, and I am excited to discuss it with you, but first, can you tell me why you decided to become a Chiropractor?

I began the arduous and dedicated process of becoming a doctor when I was five years old. There was an educational demonstration presented by uniformed nurses from the local Red Cross whose purpose was to inspire youngsters to join the medical field, and I felt a calling!

I returned from school that day and informed my mother that one day I will become a doctor. Of course, like many mothers, she was thrilled. She gave me a big hug, smiled at me with encouraging eyes and said, "You will be a great doctor one day!"

I had not learned until later in my life that my mother suffered a terrible tragedy earlier in her life when a Chiropractor could have saved her from a month of unimaginable anguish. On the day of her 16th birthday before she was to attend her sweet 16 party she sneezed while bent over tying her shoes and her back seized in a fully bent over position. At the same time, her first menses uncomfortably surprised her. Doctors were baffled, and she was placed in a full body cast for a month until enough muscles atrophied allowing her to move again. I believe that it was this traumatic experience that coalesced into a seed in my mother's psyche for a child to be born (me) that could help prevent this from happening to others in the future.

As for deciding to become a Chiropractor in my personal timeline through my own experience, it was the last type of doctor that I thought I would become because I heard from an early age that Chiropractors are not real doctors.

Following four years of pre-medical studies at Goucher College, Baltimore, MD, the sister school to Johns Hopkins, I was surprised to discover that I was disenchanted with not only the process of applying to medical school, but the with the western medical profession entirely. I shadowed surgeons for 100 hours as an internship. I found their daily routine to be boring and mundane. They performed the same surgeries over and over with little encouragement or opportunity to express creativity.

Another promising internship brought me to Philadelphia, The City of Brotherly Love, or rather of pipe bombs under cars, violent muggings, and other atrocities that frightened this country bumpkin who grew up on a mountain with only four neighbors. On the bright side, Philly boasted beautiful brick row houses, charming, narrow cobble stone streets and rich American History. There, I conducted laboratory research in the Children's Hospital of Pennsylvania creating an oral vaccine to Rotavirus. I enjoyed this type of work and believed that if I could innovate a cure in a lab then I could help more people than I could working one-on-one as a surgeon or as a clinician.

Following my graduation from the beautiful stone buildings and green rolling hills painted with equestrian and lacrosse champions at Goucher College, I moved to the Biotech Bay, San Francisco, CA where I learned the startling truths of the goings on in corporate cancer research start-ups. Initially inspired to innovate and heal the masses, I became disheartened during my four years in corporate labs to learn that the bottom line was actually profits at any cost. I experienced enough embezzlement, fraud, back stabbing and espionage to write a movie that could rival *Downloaded*, which vividly depicts the roller coaster rise and fall of the first Internet-based music sharing app., Napster.

Inspired by the teachings in the Yoga Sutras of Patangali by the late, great B.K.S. Iyengar, I decided that I wanted to begin a more virtuous path more true to my values by working with clients one-on-one in a holistic health field. So in 2001 I began learning every type of rehabilitative massage therapy, energy work, etc. that I could. I soon built a thriving injury rehab practice where I received referrals from local Chiropractors, Osteopaths, Medical Doctors, and a host of Holistic Practitioners with whom I regularly networked.

When did you decide to make knees your specialty?

Following my training in Hendrickson Method (www.hendricksonmethod.com) is when I heard my calling as a knee specialist. This method involves the combination of cross fiber massage strokes, joint mobilizations and manual resistive techniques for the correction of various soft tissue injuries, which we were taught to assess. Dr. Tom Hendrickson told us about how he healed his own meniscus tear by receiving his method from a colleague, receiving Chiropractic adjustments and practicing knee circles, a Tai Chi / Kung Fu warm-up exercise.

Shortly after I learned how to do Hendrickson Method and that it could be a helpful part of healing knee injuries, a Chiropractor sent me my first client referral with a knee joint-locking problem. I applied what I learned from Dr. Hendrickson and the joint locking problem resolved. This patient also suffered from a tendinitis in her knee, which she suffered from for many years. She believed it was permanent because this is what she was told by her MD. I applied my skills from the Hendrickson Method, namely cross fiber friction to the painful, damaged area which stimulates tears to heal and had the patient gently contract and relax the muscles on each side of the joint back and forth which increases circulation to the area and eliminates muscle imbalances across the joint. After a few office visits where I repeated the Hendrickson Method techniques specific to the patient's assessment, the pain subsided and full function was restored. As others in the Bay Area learned what I could do I began to receive additional referrals with knee complaints, and I continued to have success at helping them to heal without the need for drugs or surgery.

I went on to learn other techniques to help my patients as I began to receive more and more complex cases.

What kind of knee injuries do you treat?

As long as the knee joint is not completely dismembered, I seem to be able to help. I've returned patients in wheel chairs and those whom require crutches and canes as well as those with all manner of combinations of the following to return to active sports and normal daily activities:

- Meniscus tears

- Ligament sprains (ACL, PCL, MCL, LCL)

- Menisco-capsular sprains

- Joint capsule sprains

- Joint locking

- Lateral patellar tracking dysfunction

- Severe cartilage loss

- Muscle atrophy

- Tendonitis

- Bursitis

- Enthesopathy

I have even helped patients with 20+ years of chronic pain. It's not always possible to get the patient 100% pain free when they wait too long to come in because too much of the actual structures are destroyed. Even still the patients are typically overjoyed to have significantly less pain or even some days without any pain at all.

How soon should someone come to see you if they have a knee injury?

Anyone concerned with or without pain and injury is welcome to come in to be evaluated. According to research, most knee injuries begin with chronic destruction of the knee joint which weakens the supporting structures like the meniscus and the ACL. There may be no pain associated with this process. Then, a single traumatic event occurs like a sudden stop or a twist of the knee. It may not even be that severe of a single stop or a twist. It is just that final motion that tore that final set of fibers that were holding the meniscus or the ACL together. You know that phrase, "The straw that broke the camel's back?" It's like that. So, I can see that coming with a combination of imaging studies like X-Ray and MRI and by taking a health history and performing a physical exam consisting largely of range of motion assessment, muscle strength testing and other orthopedic and neurologic testing.

Isn't it bad for a patient with a meniscus or ligament tear to postpone surgery?

Many sports medical doctors/orthopedists now recommend waiting a period of time (1 - 2 months) to see if the injury will heal on its own before preforming any surgery. Many recommend physical therapy during this time. Just waiting sounds negligent to me. Why not correct the underlying motion disturbance pattern in the body that made the knee joint susceptible to injury in the first place? This will in turn set the stage for the knee to heal itself.

To me waiting to see if something will heal is like telling someone with a car engine problem to just wait it out. I'd rather take the car to an appropriately knowledgeable mechanic who can fix the problem. Now if I suspect it's an alignment problem, should I take my car to an oil change service station? No, the correct solution is to take the car to a specialist with training that is commensurate with the complexity of the suspected malady, get it diagnosed correctly and fixed accordingly. This is also the case with a physical injury like a knee injury.

Following an exhaustive review of the available literature in peer reviewed journals dating back almost 100 years in order to prepare for my recently published case study, I found that non-surgical, conservative management of meniscus tears, the most common injury of the knee joint, is currently the preferred method of intervention over surgery due to the observation of negative long-term clinical results associated with the removal of part or all of this important structure.

Does it not make sense to correct the biomechanics i.e. how the body moves, prior to repair of the structures that were damaged in the body due to the faulty biomechanics? For example, if a car is driven with poor alignment then the tires wear unevenly. Over time the tires show visible signs of wear such as steel radial fibers being exposed. Then, if under high speeds, sharp curves and/or a sudden stop, the tire may blow out. Now, is the solution to just patch the tire or replace the tire or fill the hole in the tire with a resinous matrix? Or, should we correct the alignment, the problem that is compromising the integrity of the tire, then address the damage to the tire? Yes, the alignment should be corrected, then various methodologies may be considered for addressing the damage to the tire; otherwise, the tire is simply going to blow out again. The same is true of knee injuries. If you try to surgically repair part of the knee without correcting the underlying motion disturbance patterns that are compromising its form and function, then the surgery is likely to fail.

So, surgery is never needed for meniscus tears?

Following an evidence-based care model, which is the gold standard of modern medicine, the correct answer is that surgery should be avoided initially and a conservative approach to care is recommended, i.e. what I do, unless the knee injury involves a root tear or a radial tear of the meniscus.

Why are those types of tears so important?

A root tear pulls the meniscus from the bone where it attaches, and a radial tear is a tear within 1cm of where it attaches. Both of these types of tears render the meniscus ineffective at its myriad functions. Having this type of tear would be akin to having no meniscus at all. Joint degeneration would ensue quickly and likely necessitate joint replacement surgery.

Surgeons have been reattaching these types of tears in hopes of preserving the function, but unfortunately according to the current literature most of these actually fail. Again, the surgeons are not recommending correcting biomechanics first, then they are baffled why the surgeries fail.

Let's go back to our example of the car with an alignment problem. This would be like putting a new tire on a car with an alignment problem and then wondering why the tire blew out again in a short amount of time.

Some people are confused by this analogy so I will make another one. A door hung on its hinges incorrectly digs a hole in the floor. Then the homeowner replaces the floor only to wonder why when the door swings open and closed again it digs a hole in the floor. Is the correct solution to fill the hole in the floor again? How about fill the hole with pain pills? Perhaps the floor is deficient in pain pills? No, the door must be hung correctly, and then the floor must be repaired.

The research studies I've reviewed dating back to 1923 offer little explanation as to why some knee injuries heal on their own while others do not. It is not known why some surgeries are successful and others do not resolve the patient's pain. And, there is little explanation as to why physical therapy helps sometimes and why many times it does not. The case studies I am currently publishing are of great significance, as they will be used as examples to explain the underlying mechanism that predisposes the knee to injury and the subsequent role this mechanism plays in the inability of many knee injuries to heal.

Will you do other research?

I will continue to publish case studies demonstrating the efficacy of my work, and I am currently planning further research making use of wearable goniometers, joint range of motion measuring devices, as well as wearable joint pressure sensors and advanced digital gait analysis imaging to both quantify and qualify the safety and efficacy of my methods.

You sure know a lot about healing knee injuries...

It is difficult to truly get everyone to understand what I understand about healing injuries due the complexity of how motion disturbance patterns hide in the body. It's sort of like asking a software engineer to explain how to make a piece of computer software such as Microsoft Word, but I will do my best to explain the important general process that makes my work so successful.

Most cases of knee pain need to be assessed for soft tissue injury and myofascial shortness weakness vs. neuro-segmental joint dysfunctions as well as contributing cranial/visceral/meningeal torsion and tension patterns, and associated organ reflex dysfunctions and their resultant muscle weakness patterns. These are the most common predisposing factors to knee pain and injury or any injury in the body of biomechanical origin, and they are oftentimes intricately biomechanically coupled affecting full body kinematic chains of muscle and fascia. For example, cranial bone motion is coupled with foot and ankle motion such that an ankle sprain may prove difficult to fix without first normalizing cranial bone motion. Similarly, motion may need to be normalized at the fourth lumbar vertebrae as well as through the sacroiliac joint in order to normalize motion through the knee joint.

Much less often emotional/psychological, nutritional/toxicity/ rheumatological complicating factors, and significant muscle atrophy play a role the patient's ability to heal from a knee injury. The vast majority of my knee patients whom I have been treating since 2001 recover from their severe knee injuries without having to do any physical therapy exercises other than knee circles.

Can you put that a little more simply perhaps?

Sure. A body not moving well for various reasons causes more wear and tear on certain structures in the body and it is super easy to recognize and manage by a properly trained therapist or doctor.

So, is physical therapy good for knee injuries?

Perhaps the standard medical approach consisting of physical therapy prior to surgery hopes to address this all-important issue of faulty alignment and biomechanics. Unfortunately, the current state of most physical therapy approaches lack the specificity and comprehensiveness necessary to adequately address this goal.

Most physical therapy these days involves strengthening weak muscles. Now, if the muscle is testing weak due to an underlying neuro-segmental joint dysfunction (a situation where the brain has lost proper control of a joint and it moves incorrectly, weakens muscles, and causes or perpetuates pain, inflammation and destruction of tissues) for which I can correct in a single office visit to restore near 100% muscle strength and near 100% normal range of motion, then does it make sense to instead enroll a patient into 6 weeks of physical therapy to attempt to achieve the same goal that I can accomplish in a single office visit? The answer is no. In addition, the physical therapy may make the injury worse if there is also a motion disturbance pattern causing uneven forces through the joints of the body. Let's recall the example of a door hung on the hinges incorrectly digging a hole in the floor. Exercising the dysfunctional joint is akin to opening and closing the door repeatedly and hoping the door alignment will fix itself.

In support of physical therapy, I will mention that there is very good evidence in the literature to suggest that patients can strengthen their way out of their maladies. Physical therapy may be helpful if there is significant muscle atrophy but only after spinal neuro-segmental dysfunctions and cranial distortion patterns are corrected which cause the bulk of muscle weaknesses and imbalances; otherwise, the patient is fighting an uphill battle as they are being asked to fight neurologic inhibition of muscles unnecessarily. Remove neurologic inhibition first with cranial and Chiropractic adjusting, directly repair tissue tears with cross fiber friction, treat fascial shortenings, which clearly cause significant muscle weaknesses, with myofascial release therapies, then instruct patients to stretch what is short and tight, then strengthen what is weak with appropriate exercises. This is the correct order of operations.

What caused the door or more importantly the person to get out of alignment in the first place?

Being born, learning to walk, playing sports, not sitting, standing or moving correctly all contribute to muscle imbalances with cause uneven forces through the joints, which is a primary cause of joint destruction.

Why do you say, "Fascial shortenings clearly cause significant muscle weaknesses?" What does that mean?

Fascia is the connective tissue made of tiny fibers that cover muscles like the skin on a sausage. If the fascia gets bunched up or stuck to the muscle it can cause a severe weakness. If you look at or touch the given muscle with a significant fascial shortening you can clearly see that it is not atrophied; however, when challenged against resistance it tests very weak. A patient may not be able to hold up their leg, or perhaps their leg buckles under their weight when they try to stand. If the practitioner can isolate the muscle(s) with the fascial shortening and then stretch it with massage like strokes, then the patient can immediately see a dramatic improvement in muscle strength.

I was recently treating an NFL player who could not sit on the exam table with his knees bent and his feet flat on the table and his arms crossed as if doing a sit up. He would fall backwards from apparent muscle weakness. Did he need to go to physical therapy? Clearly he had huge, solid, bulbous muscles. I stretched the fascia overlying his abdominal muscles, and immediately his muscle strength was increased such that he could sit up and resist all the force I could muster. He was astounded!

This is because the muscles exert their force through the fascia. If the fascia becomes shortened then the muscle will clearly test weak.

Now imagine the Chiropractor who does not assess and treat the fascia.

Imagine one who thinks the joints alone can be manipulated to correct all manner of maladies. Their treatments are likely to fail or to take much longer because they did not fully assess and treat specifically a given aspect of the patient's diagnosis.

What are some of the predisposing factors that cause knee injuries?

Janette Travell who wrote the giant Trigger Point books mentioned that the most common problem in the body that predisposes it to injury is an adhesion in the body, i.e. an area of the body that is stuck together. She goes on to mention that the most common cause for an adhesion in the body is another adhesion in the body.

An adhesion in one part of the body causes more motion to occur somewhere else in the body. This additional motion somewhere else puts a strain on the muscles, tendons, ligaments, joints in that area predisposing it to injury similar to the analogy mentioned earlier involving a door hung unevenly on its hinges and digging a hole in the floor.

Then, as that area of the body experiences micro trauma, the body reflexively tightens muscles around that area in order to protect it from further injury. This causes more motion to happen in another area of the body and the sequela continues.

Adhesions can hide anywhere in the body such as within the muscles, within the fascia, within the joints, within the cranial sutures, between body organs, within nerve sheaths, etc. Each area needs to be assessed and addressed with the appropriate, specific technique. Massage/myofascial modalities like Hendrickson Method, Active Release Technique, etc. work well on these.

Left uncorrected for long enough, the adhesions cause neuro-segmental joint dysfunctions also called subluxations. The word neuro-segmental joint dysfunction describes a joint that is not being controlled correctly by the brain, which results in marked muscle weakness in one or more muscles in that area, altered joint motion in that area and even increased signaling in the sympathetic nervous system which may contribute to chronic illness. Chiropractic techniques work well on these. I prefer to work primarily with Activator Methods Chiropractic Adjusting due to its specificity in a framework of Sacro-Occipital Technique because it appreciates the nature of how cranial bone misalignments, restrictions within the coverings of the nervous system, and organ reflex dysfunctions can prevent chiropractic adjustments from having adequate efficacy.

The progression of adhesions and the resultant aberrant body motion compensations to avoid pain and protect joints is variable and insidious. The managing practitioner must be astute and well trained in multiple modalities in order to effectively identify the exacting restriction that is to be corrected in the correct order for that specific patient receiving treatment in order for treatment to be effective.

Understanding all this, is it no wonder that it may seem impossible for some people to heal from their injuries or for most doctors to be baffled as to the cause of a patient's pain or inability to heal? It's complex. It can be really, really, really darn complex.

To make things worse there can be complicating factors to healing such as comorbidities, i.e. diagnoses such as high blood pressure or diabetes. Some prescription medications can even cause muscle and joint pains or inabilities to heal.

So when someone asks me if there is some exercise or some stretch they can do my response is this: I need to take a complete patient history, do a complete exam, study imaging reports from X-Ray and MRI. Then, I typically need to correct some motion restriction patterns with any of 30 techniques over the course of 5 – 15 office visits. Then,

I can give the patient some exercises or stretches if necessary. Otherwise, suggesting a regimen of stretches or strengthening seems negligent. It would not be the correct thing to do.

Can you tell me more specifically how these altered motion patterns in the body predispose someone to a knee injury specifically?

Most certainly, the locomotor system of the human body is largely composed of fibers including muscles, tendons, ligaments and fascia. Muscles have contractile fibers and the contraction of their fibers exerts a force on the fibers of the fascia, which are coverings of the muscles and fibers that connect all of the parts of the body together to help it to move much the same as the strings of a marionette move a puppet. Go ahead and attach some of the strings of a marionette together and watch how the motion of the puppet is disturbed.

Here is a more specific example. In just about all of my knee patients, perhaps all of my knee patients, they have a functional short leg. Now this is not an anatomical short leg. They have one hip that is rolling forwards, one rolling backwards, and a muscle imbalance that permeates their entire structure perpetuated by a series of neuro-segmental joint dysfunctions, myofascial shortenings, adhesions and/or tiny tears of fascia, and a cranial distortion pattern. This causes one hamstring to be shorter and tighter than the other. The hamstring fascia near the knee is continuous with the meniscus and responsible for its proper motion when the knee bends. Long term, this misalignment pattern pulls and tugs unevenly on the meniscus and possibly the other ligaments of the knee like the ACL damaging it with micro tears and preventing it from healing. Then, one day the patient makes that one final motion that tears the last remaining fibers holding the structure together.

That sounds like it makes so much sense. How come sports medical doctors are not doing anything about this?

I must say that I don't know. It baffles me. The apparent disparity of hip flexion when comparing right to left is obvious. With the patient lying on their back and flexing one hip with the leg held straight, the practitioner can feel how far the hip flexes and the relative tension of the hamstring muscle group on the back of one leg. Then if you compare that to the other leg, the properly trained practitioner can easily tell that one flexes well with a springy end feel and the other stops way short and feels rather rigid at its end range. This is common and it is not normal, and it is what largely predisposes the knee and other structures such as the hip or shoulder to injury. When comparing the left and right sides of the body, the joints of the body should have relatively uniform flexion and extension, and the muscles should have uniformly springy end feels at the end of each joint range of motion. A joint with reduced range of motion and muscles with rigid end feel is a ticking time bomb, and they should certainly not be present in the professional athlete or in the professional dancer.

Can't the person just stretch the short tight muscle?

Great question! The answer is a resounding, No! I worked as a very well trained massage therapist for ten years prior to studying Chiropractic. I know how to loosen any muscle or tissue in the body by a number of methods. It is absolutely detrimental to try to stretch out a muscle that is being actively inhibited by a cranial or neuro-segmental joint dysfunction (subluxation). Oh how I have tried, and oh how I have failed.

It is completely ignoring the power of our nervous system. Sadly, it creates more slack in the system to tighten up around the joint that needs to be adjusted. My baffled yoga teacher patients will tell you this.

They are in awe when I show them how the correct joint adjustment allows the muscles to lengthen, increasing joint range of motion significantly without any stretching.

Is it possible to naturally heal a damaged knee joint without surgery?

It happens every day. There is a recent review article that tells of ACLs repaired surgically where the meniscus tear was left untreated. Of those left untreated 50% - 61% of medial menisci and 55% - 74% of lateral menisci showed complete healing upon follow-up arthroscopy or arthrography. The surgeons reported that this rate of healing is poor and that more surgeries are needed. It is my belief that these rates are excellent, and that all of these patients need their biomechanics diagnosed and improved preoperatively to see if a surgery is even necessary. Then, if surgery is necessary then they still need biomechanical rehabilitation pre and post operatively from a well-trained Chiropractor. The Chiropractor is the only professional adequately trained to identify and correct neuro-segmental joint dysfunctions, which are a major part of most injuries.

My treatment *Active Knee Care*^{TM} is the most comprehensive approach to not only knee joint healing but to entire body motion restoration and function because Active Knee Care^{TM} includes a method to identify maladapted motion patterns in the body and to neutralize them. This creates the ideal environment for the body to heal itself.

What makes Active Knee Care™ the best treatment for healing knee injuries?

Active Knee Care^{TM} is the most well thought out conservative management plan for various knee joint diagnoses because it correctly identifies a multitude of various associated diagnoses present in the entire body and clears them in the correct order and with the most relevant manual therapy modality. It is a method of identifying and correcting motion disturbance patterns anywhere in the body, which contribute to uneven forces in the knee joint. It is these uneven forces through the knee joint that predispose the knee to injury and prevent it from healing. Any restriction in the body affecting the knee must be identified, neutralized and corrected. The patient must receive treatments until the legs become equal length when examined face up as well as face down on the exam table. All muscles in the body must test strongly to resistance, and patients who can and will practice my knee circles exercise progressively up to hundreds of times a day show the best outcomes.

How many office visits does it take?

The answer to that question is similar to a patient asking their dentist when they can remove their braces. The answer they will likely receive is that they can have their braces removed when their teeth are straight. Likewise, we can cease treatments or move to a maintenance program of office visits less often when symptoms are thoroughly under control or are eliminated completely and the leg length is equal face up as well as face down on the exam table. Younger patients with recent injuries whom are active without complicating factors may only require a single office visit for a meniscus tear. Older patients with severe degeneration and complicating factors may require as much as 3 months of consecutive office visits before they reach their maximum medical benefit from Active Knee Care™.

Most patients show a complete resolution of pain, or the more difficult cases choose to live with their considerable improvement and small amount of residual/intermittent pain or they move onto surgeries such as meniscus repair, ACL restoration, partial or full joint replacement.

Some knee injuries cause a lot of swelling. Don't they need surgery if they have extreme swelling and they cannot move their knee at all?

Many surgeons will not perform surgery on a very swollen knee that lacks full extension. Active Knee Care™ does an excellent job of restoring the fullest range of motion possible and decreasing joint swelling. If a patient must move onto surgery they will have optimized outcomes because their joint motions are corrected as much as possible, swelling is decreased or eliminated and complicating factors are neutralized as much as possible. In addition, patients are thoroughly educated as to why their injury occurred and what to do to identify or to correct problems that pop up in the future. Following surgery, Active Knee Care™ should be resumed for an applicable period of time.

Can you tell us about a patient who was able to cancel their knee surgery because of you?

There are many; although, the most entertaining perhaps is the man I approached in a wheel chair who told me that if I could fix his knee then he would buy me a car. His story is captured on my YouTube channel and on my website. See www.youtube.com/drdavidsundy I restored 100% of his function, he cancelled his surgery, and he bought me a matchbox car.

Did you ever experience any feedback from a knee surgeon?

I met in person with a local Sports Medical Orthopedist regarding my work and she was fascinated. She offered to play an active role in my continued research. The study I am planning next will involve wearable technology to measure changes in joint angles and pressures as patients progress through care in order to quantify the relevant improvements and to validate that it is in fact my treatment that is accomplishing the improvements in normalizing joint motion and pressures.

Do you only work with athletes or also regular folks from all walks of life?

I've treated all manner of folks large and small, young and old, NFL to weekend warrior. It is much easier to treat professional athletes as they follow all of my recommendations, show up to all of their appointments, and then they achieve excellent results. Moms and youngsters also keep their appointments and show excellent results. The busy professionals are difficult to treat. They have a lot of stress and they tend to miss appointments often. They usually do not have time to do rehabilitative stretches and strengthening exercises and they often ask when they will be better like a child in the backseat of a car during a road trip asking, "Are we there yet?" I tell them that they have to actually show up for their appointments and they need to follow my recommendations. Many corporations are now creating wellness centers with Chiropractors, Massage Therapists, Acupuncturists, etc. on site to serve this busy population whom is best served by someone who can treat them in between meetings and work. They simply do not have time before, during or after work to make it in regularly for treatments.

Is there anything that people can do to prevent knee problems?

Since most knee injuries are the result of cumulative micro trauma caused by uneven hips and a functional short leg, people should get checked regularly by a qualified Chiropractor who checks leg length and can make them equal whether the patient is being checked on an exam table lying face up or face down. Both are important. All of my patients who eventually develop even leg length show the best outcomes.

What type of Chiropractic do you receive?

There are well over 120 different types of Chiropractic modalities. My favorite type of chiropractor is a SOT doc, a Sacro-Occipital Chiropractor or Craniopath. It's a technique created by a doctor who was a mechanical engineer, an Osteopath and a Chiropractor.

They know how to correct cranial bone and meningeal (coverings of the nervous system) restrictions and adhesions. They also know how to clear organ reflex patterns, organs stuck in nervous system feedback loops causing or perpetuating muscle pain as well as organ dysfunction. Left untreated, both of these can make Chiropractic adjustments ineffective. The doc should also check joint motion in all joints of the body before and after each office visit and they should practice Activator Methods Chiropractic adjusting because it makes use of objective not subjective tests to check where an adjustment should be made and whether it was effective. In addition, they should know how to clear myofascial restrictions and how to repair tissue tears with cross fiber friction massage. However, I do not know anyone else other than myself who does all of this in a single office visit as most docs are simply not trained in this many techniques and it is rather time consuming. It takes about 45 minutes for me to complete a thorough treatment such as this.

In addition to adjusting away all neuro-segmental joint dysfunctions (subluxations) ameliorating lower cross and upper cross syndromes is also necessary for healthy knees and other joints in the body. These are muscle imbalances that can be corrected with stretches and strengthening exercises. This is where physical therapy is needed. Without the correct PT following my treatment some patients will plateau with low-level pain and dysfunction due to muscle imbalance patterns.

What are muscle imbalances?

Muscle imbalance patterns are where muscles are short and tight on one side of a joint and stretched out and weak on the opposite side of the joint. Physical therapy is the most specific treatment for this condition once all other factors are corrected. Muscle imbalance is a specific diagnosis where physical therapy is the right tool for the right job.

Are there other exercises on your YouTube channel to help people with knee injuries?

No, because it can be detrimental to exercise with a body out of alignment. Patients should get checked first by a qualified, well-trained Chiropractor then follow the exercises specific to their condition.

My YouTube channel www.youtube.com/drdavidsundy shows a lot of patient success stories from actual patients, many of whom were able to cancel their surgeries before their surgery date.

Practicing knee circles regularly with knees and feet touching can help to stimulate healing of the structures in the knee. There is a link to this exercise on my YouTube channel.

How can people reach you?

Phone: 415-425-2859
Fax: 415-487-9226
YouTube: www.youtube.com/drdavidsundy
Website: www.activehealing-sf.com
Yelp: http://www.yelp.com/biz/david-b-sundy-dc-san-francisco
FB: https://www.facebook.com/drdavidsundy
Twitter: https://twitter.com/drsundy

Do people come to see you from outside of San Francisco?

Most definitely, some travel 1 – 2 hours from far North and from far South. Some are referrals from other doctors who researched the best possible specialist to help them. Other times these patients have tried multiple practitioners over the course of many years and then through extensive web search they learned of my knee specialty practice and extensive success at helping everyday folks as well as professional athletes such as NFL players and professional dancers.

My furthest away patient was a young lady (my sister) who was left with a paralyzed leg following a pregnancy (labor and delivery of her baby). I flew to Tucson once every couple of months to treat her. She hadn't walked for two weeks when I first examined her. I adjusted joints in her spine and cranial bones that restored muscle strength to her paralyzed leg. It was still numb, but now the muscles were firing. I taught her to walk during the initial visit with a walker, and I left her with an electric muscle stimulation device to retrain the muscles of her leg. During the next couple of months, she made only slow progress with physical therapy. I returned again to treat her and she improved markedly, gaining noticeable feeling back in her numb leg. She showed slow progress until my next treatment. Then as the feeling returned to her leg she noticed that she had a knee injury, which most likely occurred from a fall in the hospital following her delivery. I treated that two times, and that resolved. Now nearly one year later she is fully recovered. She tells me that no other treatment seemed to help her except for my adjustments and therapies.

About the Author

Dr David Sundy D.C.

Active Healing-SF
4200 18th Street, Suite 204
San Francisco, CA 94114
Phone: 415-425-2859
Fax: 415-487-9226
YouTube: www.youtube.com/drdavidsundy
Website: www.activehealing-sf.com
Yelp: http://www.yelp.com/biz/david-b-sundy-dc-san-francisco
FB: https://www.facebook.com/drdavidsundy
Twitter: https://twitter.com/drsundy

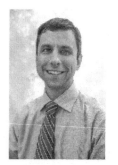

Dr. David Sundy treats patients in the San Francisco Bay Area, where he specializes in treating knee injuries primarily combining motion and functional assessments with Activator Methods, Hendrickson Method, Cranial Adjusting and Laser Therapy all in a framework of Sacro-Occipital Technique. He began his practice in 2001 as a massage therapist and graduated from Life Chiropractic College West in 2010. He learned as many modalities as possible to help his patients, and he is currently trained in 30 techniques. When he's not with his patients, publishing case studies or presenting and teaching at research symposiums he enjoys indoor rock climbing, roller skating, gourmet cooking, and hiking throughout the San Francisco Bay Area.

MULTI-GENERATIONAL FAMILY CARE

By Dr. Jeff Pereverzoff

Tell me about your practice and what kinds of patients you help?

Our practice is truly a family practice environment. We always have infants and toddlers around the office. We check many newborns within a few days of birth. My staff loves kids. I think my assistant Jennifer would tell you that carrying around the babies and playing with the toddlers is one of her favorite parts of her day.

We of course look after their parents and grandparents as well. At the other end of the spectrum there is often a walker in the reception area. Currently we have a number of patients in their 90's.

Our mission and purpose is to help people of any age express their full human potential and a state of well-being by optimizing the function of nervous system and spine. If I can help someone's nervous system function at higher level, then every aspect of their life can be better. Every body function...every interaction...everything!

There are a number of key components to health and a healthy spine and nervous system is critical... that is what we do best.

Kids who get chiropractic checkups regularly are healthier. Likewise, adults that receive regular chiropractic care are healthier.

We help families live to their full potential by teaching them how to manage the three kinds of stress....physical....chemical...and mental/

emotional.

More people are living to be 100 years of age and beyond than ever before and there is a good chance you may get there. How do you want to live those years?

What led you to this field, Dr. Pereverzoff?

Well, originally, I was going to either be a doctor or a dentist. I was treated by a chiropractor at 11 years of age for headaches and nosebleeds, and it was basically symptom-based care, which is what my family and I were looking for. Headaches and nosebleeds were awful, especially the nosebleeds. You couldn't just take a Tylenol for a nosebleed and it was quite inconvenient to say the least. My nose would just open up like a tap for no apparent reason. I didn't particularly like going to the chiropractor because I had an old-fashioned chiropractor that used to make me disrobe right down to my underwear, and the adjustments were very aggressive. However, it solved the problem.

In the following years, as I started playing golf with my father, I often crossed paths with my medical doctor at the golf course. As time went on, I played golf with my doctor once in a while, and as we started talking about career choices I said I'd like to be a doctor or a dentist, and he said, "Well, dentists have the highest suicide rate of any profession, so you don't want to be a dentist."

And he said, "I'm a medical doctor," and he continued, "and do you notice sometimes in the middle of my round of golf I get called away? And I have to go to emergency calls in the middle of the night. It's not a good lifestyle. If you want a lifestyle with a family and kids, why don't you be a chiropractor?" He knew of my chiropractic history, and that chiropractic care worked for me, and probably knew a few chiropractors and said, "It's a great lifestyle, you should take a run at it."

When I started university, I still hadn't completely committed to becoming a chiropractor. All of the requirements for sciences were the same whether it was dental, chiropractic, or other health-related studies. I knew I wanted to do something in the health-related field, so during the first couple of years of university, I talked to a lot of chiropractors and different medical doctors and professionals. The chiropractors had a much better lifestyle and many of them we very happy with their work. Many said they loved going to work every day. So I decided to become a Chiropractor and applied to several schools. I was accepted to four different schools, and ultimately it came down to California or Toronto, but the California school really catered to Canadian students. I chose the school in California and it was great. The weather was much nicer than Toronto winters for sure.

Then you decided to come back home. Did you set up your practice in Kelowna right away?

Yes, I did. I was a little bit torn because I wanted to stay in California, but the lifestyle of the San Francisco Bay area was just a bit too hectic after growing up in a small town of 3500 people. Even though we loved the beaches and the climate, I wanted to be closer to my family. Kelowna, BC, was the obvious choice; we have everything here, lifestyle-wise, and living here fits in with the whole chiropractic lifestyle of being active and enjoying balance in your life.

In your early years in your practice, did you mostly focus on symptom and crisis care, or wellness/lifestyle care?

The early years of the practice were basically symptom care. The school I went to was a little bit more symptom-based and focused on treating pain and symptoms, and was a little more medically-oriented. There is a large part of the chiropractic profession that practices in sort of a medical model, treating symptoms, whether it's back pain, neck pain, or headaches. I was an athlete, playing all the sports growing up, and so I was very active when we moved here to Kelowna. I began working with the football team and some of the other sports teams.

As a result, our practice attracted a lot of athletes, and many weekend warrior-type people. I also became a weekend warrior, playing sports on the weekends, and working during the week. That was a big part of our practice until almost seven or eight years later, when my first son was born.

Suddenly, I realized that you can't treat an infant the same way you treat an athlete or a weekend warrior. You can't apply the same kind of treatment model or type of adjustment to an infant or a toddler or a 93-year-old person for that matter. I started learning about treating different age groups. I attended numerous courses and sought out training to expand my skills to children first and then to seniors.

When my oldest son was about a year old, he had a reaction to an immunization and almost died. It was a major turning point in my chiropractic career because it really made me evaluate whether I was practicing the kind of chiropractic that really fit in with my philosophies on health. So I began to learn about alternatives to vaccination because I felt there had to be a better way to keep kids healthy. I really started to learn about a natural holistic drug-free lifestyle.

My son hasn't received any other immunizations since then, although he did have a tetanus shot, because if you step on a rusty nail, you do need to have a tetanus shot or you could die. That just isn't one you play with.

We will never know why our son got so ill from that immunization. All his life, he's had extensive health issues – everything from severe eczema, to a rare form of epilepsy, which he seems to have outgrown. Now he's an unbelievably fit, 19-year-old junior hockey player and he works out every day and has about 5% body fat. He lives a very healthy lifestyle in all aspects of his life. And, of course, he gets his chiropractic adjustments regularly. He's come through it very, very well. But as a result of that ordeal, of course we did not immunize our second son at all. He's one of the healthiest kids you've ever seen in your life. That experience was what really started my transition into the family model of chiropractic practice.

Did you go get extra training in pediatric chiropractic care?

Absolutely, you have to do that. It's one of the things that I do regularly… upgrading and improving my skills all the time. The way I practice now is drastically different from what we did in our early years. Originally, we were doing what I refer to as more traditional chiropractic: manual adjusting, snapping, popping, releasing, and restoring normal motion in the vertebrae and the spinal column.

Now we practice in more of what's called the tonal model. The nervous system has a specific tone and vibration. When we encounter mental/emotional, physical or chemical stress it changes the tone and vibration of that nervous system and that can adversely affect every single aspect of our health and body function. Think of your spinal cord like a guitar string…anchored at both ends. If you take the guitar string off the guitar and lay it on the table it has no tone and cannot vibrate in tune or at all. If you over-tighten that guitar string it vibrates out of tune or can snap. Your spinal cord and nervous system works just like that. It must vibrate at the correct tone to communicate effectively with the entire body. Ninety-nine percent of our adjustments are done with a little handheld instrument or a light finger-pressure. There's no manual snapping or popping or cracking done at all. In fact, our patients usually say they love their adjustments and often comment that they cannot believe how such a gentle adjustment can make such a difference in how they feel.

Gentle adjustment is extremely important of course, when you have someone's newborn infant in your arms. One of the biggest concerns that we encounter in talking to patients, when we suggest they bring their kids in to get checked, they always say, "How can you do that kind of adjustment on a child?" And we say, "We wouldn't do that kind of adjustment on a child." The actual treatment style needs to be customized to not only match the health crisis you might be dealing with, but the size of the person as well. The treatments are very light, and very gentle.

Let's move on to the topic of family care. What are some of the reasons that multiple generations of families come to your clinic?

If you are a parent, what do you want for your children more than anything? For me, I want my kids to be happy and healthy and then the rest is up to them. Often the first person to contact us is a family member in a state of crisis and they're looking to get some relief. Many times our patients are a little bit more health-conscious or maybe have read or heard about how bad medication is for you. They come to us because they don't want to be popping Tylenol or taking muscle relaxants on a daily or weekly basis. That's often the first contact point, and chiropractic is very, very good at relieving surface symptoms.

However, the problem with surface symptoms is this: science shows that only 15 percent of your nervous system is involved in sensory perception – that means 85 percent isn't. All of this stuff could be going on in your body, and you really don't have anything sensory-wise or symptom-based to tell you if you're healthy or not.

Patients often want to learn about how their health problems seem to have come out of nowhere. For example, they might say, "I've always had a healthy back, and all of a sudden I bent over to tie my shoe, or I sneezed, and I have this back problem that's been going on for months now… it just won't go away!'"

That's where it's really important that we go through an extensive history as well as our exam procedure. We do a detailed manual exam as well as some other computerized testing that is absolutely state of the art. We look at the nervous system and measure skin temperature patterns, surface EMG in the muscles, heart rate and skin conductance. Our measurements show us patterns that may have been there from an accident or an injury years ago, or some kind of a stressful incident, or a mental or emotional incident that they went through. There is even research now which shows trauma starts with the birth process itself, and if it's not corrected at a young age, it's just a matter of time before that initial insult to the spine and the nerve system causes a problem, whether it's as a toddler or a teen, or someone in their 30s or 40s.

Researchers have also determined that some of the most important developmental years for kids are between the ages of 2 and 6. Everything that happens to them during these ages is imprinted and embedded into their nervous system. The mental/emotional, physical, and chemical stresses are all affecting their nervous system dramatically. So if you have kids between 2 and 6, these are critical years for their development.

Can you talk more about the 85 percent of nerves that we have no sensory perception of?

Yes, a good example would be in the case of cancer. Cancer's not detectable when it's the size of the head of a pin. It's detectable when it's the size of your fist, or the size of a grapefruit. By then, it's already either potentially spread, or it's causing problems because now the disease process has gotten severe enough that it actually starts to alert that 15 percent of the nerve system that is responsible for sensory perception. With a lot of the state of the art technology that we utilize in our exam procedures, and with our patients that are on lifestyle programs, when we monitor them to see how they're doing, we can detect a lot of these changes in the nervous system that we couldn't detect before just by simply asking somebody how they feel. Just because you feel really good, it doesn't necessarily mean you're healthy. I think many people are starting to understand that. Waiting for symptoms to show up is not a healthy way to live.

You have a number of three- and four-generation families in your practice. Can you talk about one of these families and how they came to you?

Yes, I can tell you about our four generational family. We started with the mom. She had classic low back pain that she'd had since she had her first child 14 years prior. Over time, looking after that child and working and having a second child and not being able to exercise as much as she should, her back just got worse and worse. By the time she came to see us she was having regular spasms where she'd be laid up for three or four days at a time. We started to work with her, getting her functioning so that those spasms rarely occurred, and teaching her about chiropractic and healthy lifestyle choices.

The next step was treating her husband. He had been in a car accident, and his treatment was also symptom-based. Next we saw her mom, who had been a nurse for 40 years. She had undergone the emotional stresses of life and work along with the physical stresses of working in a physical occupation. She was having some upper back pain and some shoulder issues, and was sometimes getting light-headed and dizzy. She was really not able to work as much as she still needed to. We started working with her, and then in chatting with her, she mentioned her mother--so this is Great-Grandma now--who was 92 when we started with her. She had the typical hunched over little-old-lady posture, and was having severe upper back pain, to the point to where she really wasn't that interested in living anymore.

When Great-Grandma first came in she had her daughter on one arm and her granddaughter on the other, and she could barely walk. She couldn't even stand erect enough to look me in the eye. Our examination suggested that we might be able to do something for her, and we started adjusting her three times a week with our handy little instrument. Within a matter of a few months, her posture started to correct. Within six months, she walked in here on her own! She still uses a walker as a precaution, but she now stands almost fully erect, smiles, and can have a conversation. It's changed her life completely.

Her grandkids also come to see us. One of them suffered from panic attacks. It's interesting to note that in that family, the grandkids and Grandma have very similar forward-head, hunched-over posture.

Incidentally, this is absolutely the most common thing that we deal with because there are so many health issues related to forward-head posture. In children it can show up as hyperactivity, ADHD, allergies or asthma, and in adults it's things like heart disease and diabetes and breathing issues.

All of these different ailments have been scientifically linked to forward-head posture. You very rarely see a really healthy senior with bad posture. People in their 70s, 80s, and 90s that are in good health almost always have good posture. There is such a strong link between the health of the spine and nervous system and overall health. When you lose those spinal curves, the nervous system can't do what it needs to do, and it can affect any aspect of your health.

Forward head posture is the body's natural response to stress... mental/emotional, physical, or chemical. Think about what happens when a dog is threatened. Tail and tailbone tucks under. Think about what happens when you are startled...head and shoulders hunch down and forward. This posture puts tension on that spinal cord which then changes the tone or vibration of the nervous system. The body's response is to tighten muscles...the fight or flight response...and produces all the bad hormones and neurotransmitters. That is how stressful situations can lead to things like high cholesterol and high blood pressure.

So when we see these forward head postures we often think it is from years of sitting at a desk or computer or kids using cell phones. In reality, it is much more likely from some mental emotional stressor causing that forward head shift in response to the body's reaction to stress.

What are some of the health issues that your patients have?

Most health issues are symptoms and can be linked to nervous system dysfunction. They are your body's way of letting you know that something has gone wrong. The danger is that once you start to feel that particular health issue it has already been going on for a while.

People present to our practice with a wide variety of health issues, such as:

- Poor posture/forward head posture

- Stress symptoms and associated health issues like anxiety/headaches/poor sleep

- Weight loss and nutrition challenges

- Neck pain/shoulder pain/tingling and numbness in the hands

- Back pain/sciatica

- Depression/anxiety/hyperactivity/ Adhd

- Weakened immune system

- Ear infection/colds/flus

- Colic

- Bedwetting

- PMS symptoms/menopause

- Migraine and tension headaches

- Anxiety, depression, pain related to cancer treatment and recovery

And the list goes on...

Can you describe forward head posture?

Yes. Normally if you look at your spine from the side, it should have a very gentle S-shaped curve. There is a little curve in the neck, and then the opposite curve through the mid-back, and then the same curve in the lower back as in the neck, and then the tailbone and pelvic part of the spine again reverses the other way. A person is said to have forward-head posture if their ears are way out in front of their shoulders.

If you take a picture of your posture from the side, and you draw a gravity line from the top of the skull it should pass thru the ear canal then the shoulder then the hip and finally the ankle.

We have a posture test that we use in our initial exams, and we often send patients home with the test, saying, "Here's the posture test – do it with your family, get everybody together in the room, and have a look at each other." It is fairly easy to see when a person's head has shifted out in front of their body.

Another very important thing we look for is a tilt to the head, shoulders, or hips. You see, the spinal cord is attached to the spine like a guitar string…at the top and the bottom. This allows it to vibrate at the correct frequency to transmit nerve impulses to the entire body. If you take a guitar string and place it on a table, what does it do? Nothing! It is slack and has no ability to vibrate and make a sound. So when the body encounters one of the three stresses and the head shifts forward it stretches that spinal cord which changes the tone or vibration and now the nervous system cannot send impulses as it needs to. The body now has to compensate and ease that spinal cord tension which is does by tilting the head, shoulders, or hips. So these tilts are signs that the body has created spinal cord tension patterns that eventually cause some kind of sign or symptom. It could be something like back pain, herniated disc, or neck pain or it can be things like high blood pressure or high cholesterol.

Another issue that you work with is stress relief and associated health issues like anxiety, headaches, or poor sleep. How do you help people with that?

There are three kinds of stress: physical, chemical and mental-emotional. Physical stresses can be things like being in a car accident or a child having a sports injury, or even the birth process itself can be a physical stress on both the mother and the baby.

Secondly, chemical stresses are things in our environment like food additives, artificial sweeteners, and pollutants in the air, household toxins, and cleaners. One of the most detrimental chemical stresses is immunization but that topic would require an entire book on its own.

Finally, there is mental-emotional stress. Mental-emotional stress is so important. In fact, researchers and experts are suggesting that upwards of 80 percent of what goes wrong with your body through the course of your life is due to mental-emotional stress. Mental-emotional stresses are often manifested in physiological patterns. When adults are stressed, their shoulders pull up and pull forward, their spine wants to curl up, and it goes into almost a fetal-type position. Those stress patterns, of course, now add tension to the spinal cord and take the spine out of its normal curvatures. This position I've described is how the body protects itself, and over time it causes your spinal curves to change. This means that what your body considers a normal posture now is not normal with respect to function. It's a compensation to some sort of a stressful event.

Most people do not realize that any kind of stress: physical, chemical, or mental/emotional creates a neuro-chemical response in the body. That means it causes the body to produce things like cortisol or adrenalin which affects the entire body. That is the mechanism for mental stress causing things like high blood pressure and diabetes and obesity. It is also important to remember that the body will convert mental or chemical stress into physical stress or pain as a coping mechanism because physical stress is the least negative form. This is how mental stress can bring out things like back pain or sciatica or stiff neck.

So chiropractic care can obviously help patients with the physical issues. Do you also teach your patients about the chemical and mental stressors that are in their life?

Absolutely. That's part of what we cover when we first meet with a new patient. We discuss their history, and we can identify if their health issue is a result of a physical stressor, chemical stressor, mental-emotional stressor or all of the above.

Chemical stressors are probably the easiest to deal with. If someone has a very poor diet and eats a lot of things with artificial sweeteners and processed foods, they can easily change that. Obviously if someone's a smoker, they should stop smoking. If the patient doesn't have access to a good water source – for example if they are drinking tap water which is full of chlorine (which is toxic) – we can change that, too. Everyone should be drinking alkalized ionized water and the machines for home are very affordable. Chemical stress is pretty straightforward.

Mental-emotional stress is tougher because the mechanism is not well understood by many chiropractors and very few physicians or people in general. Research is suggesting that most of what goes wrong with our body is related to mental/emotional stress. This is truly a new idea for most people to grasp. In a lot of cases, stresses are just simple things in everyday life, like dealing with their teenage children, their boss at work, or finances, and there's a lot of little things that we teach people about that they can work on themselves.

Obviously if we can improve the tone and function of the nerve system, chiropractic care can help people deal with mental-emotional stress. It doesn't matter if it is a newborn baby or a person in their 90's.

Activities like yoga are a great way to reduce stress because it involves both a physical component as well as a mental-emotional component. People can also keep gratitude journals. Journaling is a very, very good thing. Here is another tip: when you're driving, look in the rear-view mirror and smile six times a day. Research shows that when you smile it starts to change your blood chemistry and counteract those stress hormones almost instantly. Smiling decreases the levels of cortisol and adrenaline and other stress related chemicals. There's a lot of simple little things that we do with people in cases where we determine that their mental-emotional stress is high.

I like the idea of a gratitude journal. Sometimes when people are in pain for years and years, they can tend to be negative, so if you teach them about a gratitude journal it could actually change their entire life.

That's something that I have definitely noticed over 24 years of working with people. Anything a person can do to create positive thoughts helps. Positive creates more positive. People who are more positive definitely respond better to care. It doesn't matter if it's how we used to practice in a more manual model, or in a more tonal model like we practice now. People that have more positive energy around them definitely respond better to care.

How do you help people with weight loss and nutrition?

Nutrition is the foundation. Water is really critical, and it's staggering to me when we talk to people and discover how many people do not drink one glass of pure water a day. They drink coffee, tea, Gatorade, etc, and the bottom line is that when you take your water and turn it into coffee or tea, it's not water anymore. There are still some benefits to things like green tea, of course, which is a good antioxidant, but you need to drink water in order for your body to heal, and to eliminate waste, among other things. That's the foundation of nutrition. Of course, we try to stress to people that we need to stay away from processed foods and artificial sweeteners, which are proven to cause cancer time and time again.

A balanced diet is important, but something that I have started to follow a lot in the last few years is the concept of an acidic body environment versus an alkaline body environment. Research shows that cancer and, for that matter, almost any disease, cannot live in an alkaline environment in your body, so start drinking things like alkalized ionized water and consuming foods that create an alkaline environment.

Research shows that 75 percent of the population is obese to some degree. So that means 75 percent of my patients are obese to some degree. Even myself, I'm often carrying 10 to 20 extra pounds that just seem to show up over the course of the year. At least once a year, I have a month or so where I do a very thorough cleanse for the body, and take that extra weight off. This is a very important thing that we do with our patients because when you look at the negative potential effects on your health related to obesity, things like diabetes and heart disease are becoming epidemic. Rates are just going through the roof, and that's all preventable. So, weight loss is a big issue.

We also look at the simple things related to the spine and the nervous system. If you overload that spine and that nervous system with extra weight and fat tissue that's filled with toxins, it's impossible for the body to be healthy. So through the course of our years in practice, we've always worked with people to get to a healthy weight. We have a number of different programs that we utilize in our office; some of them are simple methods of eating, some of them are products. We do lifestyle counseling for people to help keep them on track and give them guidance, and then a lot of it is sort of fine-tuning based on lifestyle.

We recommend a full complement of vitamins and minerals and protein powders. We're able to customize what they need nutritionally, and get them really good quality products. All of the supplements that we use are from the top nutritional companies on the planet; a lot of them are naturopathic or homeopathic companies with amazing track records for using the highest-quality ingredients that you can buy.

Let's talk about multi-generations having trouble with neck pain and shoulder pain. Especially kids, because they're texting all the time, and then 30, 40-year-olds because they're at their computer all the time, and then elderly people because, if they're in poor health, they may have neck problems. So how do you help them with that?

I talked a little earlier about forward head posture. Sure, things like cell phones and computers contribute to neck and shoulder pain but they are not the cause. Remember, forward head posture comes from the body compensating for physical, chemical, or most often mental-emotional stress.

There are foundational similarities in treatment for neck and shoulder pain for different ages. Infants are a little bit different of course, because they're new to the world, and their spinal curves are just developing. They're going from a C-shape curve and the secondary curves are starting to develop. When we start with toddlers and young children, we want to maintain that normal spinal curvature whether the patient is 2 or 3 years old, or whether they're a little older and starting to get very active in sports or other activities. So all of our evaluations and our adjusting protocols and exercises that we have them do are age specific. Educating them on posture and things like backpacks, are all related to get that spinal curve as close to as normal for that person as it may be. Everybody has asymmetries in their body; it's common to have one leg that's a little longer than the other. Contrary to what most people think, the body is not symmetrical. One hand's a little bigger, one foot's a little bigger, the heart's not in the center, and all of these different things are what make each person a little different.

So all of these things need to be taken into account when we look at how we are working with that particular patient. We work in a tonal model to balance and improve the vibration of the nervous system. We work to get their spinal structure as healthy as possible so that the nervous system can do what it's supposed to do. The brain makes electrical signals, sending them down the spinal cord and out through the nerves, and then the body sends signals back, and that's how the brain knows what to do next. Every single body function is controlled by electrical impulses from the brain. By restoring those normal spinal curves, it allows that nervous system to function at as high a level as possible.

You were saying children nowadays all have cellphones; can you just teach them how to use the phones differently? We can't just say, "Don't go on your cellphone." They're all texting with their head down all the time, right? So what do you do about that?

Well, that's an interesting question. The simplest one, and I used to do this with my kids when they were a little younger, is to say, "If I catch you sitting with this head down posture, you're going to lose your phone for an hour." Well they sit up straight pretty quick! It's an educational process, and as parents, we have to nag our kids. But there's little tricks you can use, like having kids use their phone laying on their bed or laying on the floor. Because, of course, if you're laying on the floor or on your bed, your spine's pretty straight. Or, sitting upright in a chair rather than a soft sofa, like more of a dining room style of chair, where they're sitting up straight and they're holding their phone up in front of their face, rather than down all curled up in a sofa with the spine shaped like a C.

Kids don't necessarily have a lot of back pain per se, their spinal cord tension tends to manifest in different ways. Headaches are a very common one. Research shows that almost 90 percent of kids have headaches on a weekly basis. That's crazy. And a lot of it is just because there's tension on their spinal cord, which causes headaches. Other symptoms that manifest from these tension patterns are things like hyperactivity, attention deficit, asthma and allergies – all these sorts of things are all related to tension patterns in the spine.

What is the 100 Year Lifestyle, and how does it relate to treating multi-generational families?

The 100 Year Lifestyle was started by a chiropractor in Atlanta named Dr. Eric Plasker. When you look at certain populations in the world, like the Hunzas and the monks, a lot of them lived to be well over a hundred years old. Much of the cell research and genetic research that's been done indicates that the way the human body is constructed, from strictly a science standpoint, if there are no stresses, and no interferences, the average person should live to be 150.

Dr. Plasker developed what he calls the 100 Year Lifestyle which follows the principle of *healthier choices mean a healthier life*. It encompasses many things including spinal health and the nervous system health, diet, and nutrition, managing stress, exercise, and even managing your finances.

Foundational to all of that is the nervous system. If the nervous system is healthy and is free of interference, the body will express a state of well-being to its full human potential, and people will live in excess of 100 years, as their body was designed to do. So, starting with checking infants right after they're born for spinal subluxations or interferences in their nervous system, and then checking people on a regular basis through the course of their life, it's going to help that nervous system function at an optimal level, and help them express their full potential. In fact, regular adjustments for mom during pregnancy can help mom have a much healthier and relaxed pregnancy resulting in an easier delivery which translates to a better development for the baby.

When it comes to multi-generational families, research shows that people who have a healthy nervous system and spine and go to the chiropractor regularly actually see their medical doctor less, they use less medication, they're actually able to live on their own seven to ten years longer before the dreaded move to assisted living. Given that we know that people who go to a chiropractor regularly and have a healthy spine have all of these other benefits to their life, why wouldn't we start checking infants right from birth, and just check them all the way through age 100 and beyond?

What is a misconception that people have about chiropractic care?

The biggest misconception is that people assume they are healthy if they are symptom free. The cancer example that I used earlier is a classic one for that. In most cases, cancer isn't detectable when it just starts; it's detectable when the cancer becomes big enough that it actually starts to show symptoms. We don't wait to brush our teeth until one falls out, do we? Now that research is linking so many diseases and illnesses to nervous system problems, why wouldn't we try to keep that nervous system as healthy as possible and prevent the symptoms?

What makes you different from other chiropractors?

There are different kinds of chiropractors just like there are different kinds of medical doctors. Some practice in a symptom relief model. Although that is important and we do some of that as well, in my opinion that is really just applying a chiropractic adjustment in a medical model. Other chiropractors practice to restore human potential and a state of well-being by optimizing nervous system function and tone. This is really what the 100 year lifestyle and lifetime care for everyone is all about. This is what we do. Our method of assessment and adjustment is very specific. We work with the tone of the nervous system and adjustments are applied using light finger pressure or a hand-held instrument called an Integrator. The Integrator is a totally unique instrument designed for use with Torque Release Technique. Adjustments are very specific and there is no cracking or popping that is experienced with manual adjustment methods.

What is your best piece of advice for families looking for natural health solutions?

We teach them about all of the 8 key components using the word **AWWESOME** as an acronym:

1. **A**nti-oxidants through food, supplements, and water.

2. **W**ater – water is not water. Water is the foundation of life. You can't live long without water.

3. **W**eight management – upwards of 70% of the population is obese to varying degrees.

4. **E**xercise – the health benefits of exercise are numerous.

5. **S**pine and nervous system health – every single body function is controlled by your nervous system.

6. **O**xygen – not only is the quality of the air we breathe important but how we breathe is important.

7. **M**ental/emotional health – so many health issues are now linked to mental/emotional issues.

8. **E**ducation, coaching and learning – where are you getting your information about how to live a healthy lifestyle? Lifestyle care is for everyone.

How can people learn more about what you do?

My websites:

www.KelownaFamilyChiropractic.com

www.KelownaFamilyChiro.com

Our facebook page:

https://www.facebook.com/KelownaChiropractor

Come in or call me for a free consultation. I love talking to people all over the world and through my affiliations I can help people find a good chiropractor almost anywhere.

About the Author

Dr Jeff Pereverzoff

Kelowna Family Chiropractic
11-2121 Springfield Road
Kelowna, BC
250-868-1167
kelownafamilychiro.com
https://www.facebook.com/Kelowna
Chiropractor/

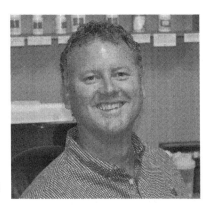

Dr. Jeff has had a family chiropractic practice in Kelowna, BC for 25 years. Kelowna Family Chiropractic has grown to be one of the largest healthcare practices in Kelowna offering lifestyle based chiropractic care, acupuncture, cold laser therapy, rolfing, massage therapy, nutritional counselling, and weight loss. Dr. Jeff graduated from Palmer College of Chiropractic West in California, with honors, and started his practice in Kelowna a few short months later.

In the early years, his practice focussed around athletes and the 'weekend warriors' as he was one himself. But, then he had his own kids and the chiropractic practice really shifted towards infants and children as well as their parents and grandparents. Dr. Jeff and Rhonda have 4 boys and he has worked with them right from birth through all stages of development and right up into their junior hockey playing days. Dr. Jeff's youngest patient was 3 days old for a routine post-birth check-up on the way home from the hospital and his oldest active patient is 94! Dr. Jeff is also affiliated with the 100 Year Lifestyle offering lifetime chiropractic care and healthy choices to help people live to 100 years of age and beyond.

Over the last 5 years, Dr. Jeff has transformed his practice with a treatment method called Torque Release Technique. This is known as a tonal chiropractic approach. The goal is to achieve better tone and balance in the nervous system thereby stimulating the body's natural healing response. This approach involves a very detailed assessment and adjustments are done by hand or by using a specially designed hand-held instrument called an Integrator. Adjustments are very light and extremely specific and patients report that it is a very comfortable adjustment. There is no manual adjusting or manipulation or "cracking" that takes place with traditional manual chiropractic treatments. His patients say that they love their adjustments!

Dr. Jeff says, "If I can help a patient's nervous system function at a higher level by removing interference…no matter what their age…wouldn't that help them in every aspect of their life?" If the nerves that control their pancreas allow it to communicate better with their brain then won't they control blood sugar better? If the nerves that control their immune system are free of interference then won't they have a stronger immune system? If the nerves that communicate with their heart communicate better with the brain then won't their blood pressure be better maintained? If the nerve system is free of interference and better able to produce hormones and neurotransmitters then won't they be able to have better interactions in every aspect of their life…at school…at work…with family members? I think you get the point!"

Dr. Jeff's mission is to provide healthy choices for families and their health care and to provide hope for patients that are struggling with their health and are 'stuck' or have not had success with traditional treatments. Whether your goal for yourself or your family is lifestyle based care and prevention or you are looking for relief from something that is limiting the things you love to do every day, Dr. Jeff can provide treatment options and care that meets your goals.

Dr. Jeff always offers a free consultation that can be done in person or by phone.

APPLIED KINESIOLOGY

By Dr. Marion Constantinides

Dr. Marion, tell me about your practice and what kinds of patients you help.

I am a natural health doctor. My doctorate is in Chiropractic and my specialty is Applied Kinesiology which allows me to practice whole body health. The people who seek me out are typically people who have had no resolution with any other type of practitioner. They may have seen multiple doctors, multiple specialists and usually I am their last hope. My patients often come to me because I am their last hope and they are truly sick and tired of being sick and tired.

What led you to this field Dr. Marion?

Originally I was on track to go to medical school. My goal was to be an emergency room physician. I had spent 12 years in the military as a combat medic and EMT. I had no issue with people having pain, but I wanted to find a way to help people stay healthy, that is what ultimately led me into chiropractic and then applied kinesiology. In chiropractic care I found a natural way for people to get well and then stay well. So instead of treating symptoms, I can help my patients live healthier.

What is applied kinesiology?

Applied Kinesiology (AK) is an advanced form of diagnosis, using the study and function of muscles to determine the best possible course of treatment for a person. The body never lies; we just have to ask the right questions in the right way to get the answer that we need to help heal the body. This is the basis of applied kinesiology.

Once we ask the right questions, we have 3 basic causes of health problems and we call that the triad of health. There is the structural, the chemical and the mental aspects. In chiropractic, mainly we are initially concerned with only the structure, as it tends to make up the base of the triangle, but all health problems, whether they are functional or pathological, are involved with one or all three of those parts of this triad. Initially my job as a Doctor who specializes in Applied Kinesiology is to determine the cause of the disease, dysfunction or pathology. Once the issue is identified, I look for the solution to the problem using manual muscle testing in conjunction with standard methods of diagnosis. A doctor who is trained in AK and understands how to properly evaluate the triad of health is able to direct treatment towards the unbalanced areas. People typically have amazing results from Applied Kinesiology.

Apart from a doctorate, what kind of training does a doctor practicing applied kinesiology require? And how long does it take?

To get the certification it is a 100 hour course and that gives you just the basics, honestly it just scratches the surface. Personally, I have taken that course three times; I have done 300 hours of supplementary training. On top of that I have completed specialized training where the purpose is to go more in depth about specific areas of the body. For example, the upper extremities, the lower extremities or the jaw are a few areas that can have a significant effect on the overall health of a person and can be addressed quickly and simply. So far, I have completed an additional 3.5-4 years post-doctoral training.

How can someone find an applied kinesiology doctor near them?

The International College of Applied Kinesiologists maintains the standards of our profession and has an online directory. Doctors who specialize in AK can be found globally at www.ICAK.com. On it you can find a doctor worldwide, it doesn't matter if you are in the US or if you are in Korea, we usually have a practitioner nearby.

What are some of the health issues that your patients have?

My patients have a myriad of issues. Often people come in initially because they have back pain. Once we start delving into their overall health a little bit further we can start finding out what the origin of the pain is: is it emotional, is it structural, is it chemical or is it toxic? Then we fix the body from there. Nobody is the same, so we don't do the same thing on every person when they come in. With each patient I complete a muscle test. I ask the proper questions to the body and through neurological and orthopedic testing, I determine how that body wants to get fixed. Sometimes it is highly specific, and sometimes it is a little bit more general.

One woman came in because she had fibromyalgia, chronic fatigue and depression. This turned out to be a misdiagnosis. For 9 years she had suffered with a multitude of debilitating disorders; she felt like an outsider looking in on her life. She would watch her husband play with the kids, she would watch them all have fun but she could never participate. It took me 6 months of working with her to determine that she had a very rare tumor in her gallbladder. She went to an oncology surgeon and had the gallbladder removed. Immediately her symptoms alleviated and she was a participant in her own life for the first time in almost ten years.

How did you notice that it was her gallbladder when no one else did?

On her first or second visit, I was able to narrow it down to the juncture between her gallbladder and her small intestine, but without an x-ray I didn't know exactly what was going on. She tested positive for parasites so I gave her some homeopathies and supplements to help kill the parasites, and that alleviated a lot of the symptoms for a short time. She got better but then after a few months she slid back again. I began to notice that the treatment I was giving her wasn't working the way that is expected with applied kinesiology. So I took a harder look at that same area and ultimately I sent her for an ultrasound of the gallbladder, and that is when the tumor was found.

Can you tell me another patient success story?

I had a patient come in with generalized back pain, who was referred by a colleague. She was a very healthy woman and had never really had any issues. As we were doing the exam, she expressed to me that she has been deaf in her right ear for about 12 years. I questioned her a little bit further, and it turns out the deafness began right after a car accident. During the accident, the right side of her head had struck the steering wheel. She was very lucky to survive that accident. Ever since then, she hasn't been able to hear out of her right ear. She has compensated by only using her left ear, turning to people when they talk; she does it really unconsciously. I tested and adjusted through applied kinesiology for a certain shift of the bones around the ear, and was able to move the bones. She regained her hearing immediately!

Have you treated anyone with breast cancer?

Yes. One particular patient had been through breast cancer twice. She was going in for another scan, and was considering a mastectomy because this would have been the third time the cancer came back. As I went through my applied kinesiology exam with her, I discovered that she had something called a neurological tooth. Not just one, she had four. Previously she had had root canals on all four of these teeth, where the mammary glands have a direct relationship with the channels or roots of these four teeth.

I sent her to a dentist to have her teeth checked, and it was discovered that her previous root canals were bad, and were in fact rotting. A root canal procedure really only gets a few of the roots from the tooth. A tooth can have over 70 channels and it is hard to get them all. She had to have two teeth removed and have a bridge placed instead. When she went back to her oncologist for her breast scan to begin treatment, they found that the cancer had spontaneously resolved.

What did the doctors say?

The oncologists said they must have been wrong, they must have got a false reading previously.

Can you help patients with depression?

Yes. I have one particular patient who suffered from depression and suicidal ideation for some time which had been progressively been worsening. She came to me because she had heard about me from a friend, a previous patient of mine who also had a debilitating disorder which I was able to successfully treat.

When treating the patient with depression I ended up using DNA testing to find that she has a few missing DNA markers in the methylation cycle. I was able to help supplement those missing areas with some simple supplements and immediately her depression alleviated; she felt like a new person. She has been able to repair her relationship with her children and her husband, who had been her number one advocate the whole time. Unfortunately, depression that is deep seeded takes a toll on the whole family. She also had a lot of anger issues, and this is a good example of how emotions can throw the body way off. She had a lot of anger from childhood injustices and we were able to work through those and help remove how those thoughts had a physiological and pathological effect on her entire organ system. Now she is feeling fantastic. With help from some simple supplements and balancing the triad, she did beautifully.

How do you help people with PTSD?

My heart really goes out to people who have post-traumatic stress disorder. Whether they are military or civilian, whatever the cause initially, their lives are forever changed. When new patients come to me with post-traumatic stress disorder I typically test their neurotransmitters first. That is a simple urine test and based on the results I can determine which specific nutritional supplements they need to boost their entire well-being. Usually I find that it is an adrenal fatigue issue, so we get their adrenals working again, and their body starts to mitigate the stress a lot better. That coupled with emotional work is the best way to remove the physical effects of post-traumatic stress disorder.

I have written a paper on stress. The body can only handle so much stress; this is based off of Hans Selye's work. I like to think of the adrenal glands as two little teacups that live on top of the kidneys. Each teacup can hold only 10 drops of stress. If you have 11 drops, the adrenal glands grow a little bit; 12 drops and it grows a little bit more. With 13 or 14 drops, the body cannot handle it any longer and it starts to secreting cortisol. At that point the adrenal glands have reached a level of demand that they cannot really come back from on their own. It causes the body to become hyper adrenal, a state where the adrenal glands are just kicking out cortisol nonstop, where your body is constantly in the 'fight or flight' mode. Eventually the adrenals will completely tap out, and stop responding. Then they are hypo adrenal, which causes many problems such as an increase of belly fat, an inability to sleep through the night, difficulty falling asleep, or an unrelenting anxiety for certain situations, which is part of the PTSD. So I strongly support the adrenal glands, which brings them back to a place where they can start to operate normally.

What is a misconception that people have about their health?

I have so many patients who come in here and they have been suffering for as little as 2 weeks to as many as 20 years with something but they all say the same thing. They all say, "You know, I really thought that this would go away." But it doesn't go away; what happens is the body begins to compensate for whatever that issue is and more pathology develops and the problem is grossly compounded.

I tell people they are bringing me their pearl of pathology. Whether it is a tiny little seed pearl if it is a new issue, or a giant pearl of Smithsonian proportions, I start peeling back the layers of that pearl until we get to that original insult, which is that tiny little bit of sand. So a patient might originally come in with stomach upset or indigestion. Once we start working through that they will have shoulder pain which they haven't had for 15-20 years, and they think that I am making them worse, but in fact we are rewinding their body through time. We are undoing all the habituation and all of compensation that has occurred from that original shoulder injury that has now caused indigestion or acid reflux.

So just ignoring things is not going to work.

No, not at all.

What is your best piece of advice for patients looking for natural help solutions?

Pain and discomfort is not a lifestyle. I love my job and I love working with people and watching when their health all of the sudden changes for the better. I think it is so important to get an applied kinesiologist near you who can help facilitate your health and your well-being. Can you imagine how great it would be to be able to rewind your clock and go back 20 years with your health and feel like you did 20 years ago? It would be miraculous! People don't have to put up with the status quo. They can really push the envelope and demand something better for themselves. That is exactly what applied kinesiology does.

How can seeking out natural health solutions help you get off medications or avoid medications all together?

My favorite example is people who take acid reducers that are proton-pump inhibitors for acid reflux, gastro-esophageal reflux disease (GERD) or chronic heart burn. People on these proton pump inhibitors are some of the sickest people who come into my office. People use them long-term but it is really only meant to be used for a short period of time. The normal course is generally to be used for only two weeks and then the patient is supposed to be re-examined. However, physicians are now prescribing proton-pump inhibitors long-term – 20 or more years – and it starts causing bone demineralization and other issues. People will take it because they have been diagnosed with acid reflux. It is so hard to get off of that. Not too long after starting the medication people may find that their body has trouble digesting, they are not absorbing any of their nutrients from their foods, they have muscle wasting, they have bone wasting and they are honestly some of the sickest people I see. People don't realize because there are joyful television commercials for these insidious drugs, which makes it appear perfectly fine and normal to both have GERD and take the drugs. To make matters worse, people are prescribing it to themselves! The drugs can now be bought over the counter inexpensively at every corner store and big chain membership clubs. It comes in a giant bottle, but people have never been told or simply do not realize that those drugs are only supposed to be for a very short term.

There is another commercial for irritable bowel syndrome right now, with a cartoon stomach and intestinal track that walk across the television. It is so bizarre.

Just watching the nightly news last night my husband and I counted 4 commercials in a row for medication. But when it comes to pain, taking medication only masks the issue. People don't realize that pain is not a lifestyle. We don't grow old and turn into painful creatures, we don't just create pain as we age. We need to take care of ourselves in order to maintain our quality of life. That is what I do more than anything. I give people back their quality of life.

How can people learn more about what you do?

I would direct them to ICAK website or ICAKUS.com. It describes what applied kinesiology is and you can find peer reviewed journal articles on there. It is just such a great conglomerate of natural health. I wouldn't choose to do Applied Kinesiology if it didn't work. You know I have really been through the gamut in my career. I have been in medicine in some form or another for 25 years at this point. It is so important to me for people to stay healthy and stay well.

About the Author

Dr Marion Constantinides B.Sc., D.C., P.A.K.

Applied Health Chiropractic
4532 Bonney road ste d
Virginia Beach, VA 23462
(757) 965-2476
www.AppliedHealthVA.com

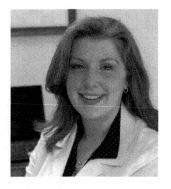

Dr. Constantinides serves her patients as individuals, educating and improving their health paradigm while supporting each person during their journey to achieving optimal wellness. She is a natural healthcare provider who uses cutting-edge, sustainable methods and specializes in assisting patients who have hard to treat health issues or have been unable to find relief through a standard course of treatment. Elite athletes and elite military who need strong, conservative (non-surgical), all natural health care also seek her services. Dr. Constantinides works diligently to quickly return people to and improved quality of life. She also works in close partnership with the Combat Wounded Coalition, providing all natural, non-medicinal and highly effective treatment to veterans with mild to severe post-traumatic stress disorder.

She is board certified in Professional Applied Kinesiology by the International College of Applied Kinesiology and in Chiropractic by the Virginia Board of Medicine. Dr. Constantinides holds her Bachelor's Degree in Biology from the University of Colorado and Doctor of Chiropractic degree from the University of Western States.

With over 25 years of experience in healthcare, Dr. Constantinides brings an extensive and unique perspective to working with all patients. As a military veteran, she has had specialty training in combat medicine and Emergency Medicine (EMT). Her military experience gives her a great deal of compassion for patients who are members of our military and their family members.

Dr. Constantinides is the author of Totally-Grain-Free.com, a blog dedicated to those with allergies and sensitivities to all grains. She has completed a documentary to illustrate how a Totally-Grain-Free lifestyle will ultimately shift the public's standard expectations of health. Dr. Constantinides is in the development stages of specialty Totally-Grain-Free products to be sold nationwide.

Dr. Constantinides volunteers with the United Way of South Hampton Roads as Vice-Chair on the Health Impact Board. The board assists non-profit organizations by designating funding for special health related community programs, as well as distributing emergency funding on an as needed basis.

She believes that education to the public and professionals is the best way to promote health. She regularly lectures to small groups in his community, at corporate events and holds education courses for special interest groups and professionals.

CHIROPRACTIC CARE FOR ATHLETES

By Dr. Victor Dolan

Sports Chiropractic History – an auspicious start

The United States has a well developed elite sports population. Name the sport, we have athletes at every level; Collegiate, Olympic, and Professional competition is front page news. We should *all* learn from these elite athletes.

These intensely competitive levels are usually played by healthy, fit, young people. Children, adolescents, and young adults are the demographic that participate in sports - people at perhaps the healthiest stage of their lives! Our elite athletes are usually between 15-35 years old, and in 'great shape'. And these 'great shape' people, super healthy, super fit, not injured, not symptomatic, not complaining - seek out Chiropractic care!

At the top levels of sport competition, a regular schedule of Chiropractic is often utilized along with the training regimen. Why would someone in the full bloom of their best health visit the Doctor of Chiropractic? Because, these athletes are seeking to improve performance even further.

Sometimes athletes resort to tactics that are not approved, and not accepted in the governing bodies of sports, and these athletes are then ostracized. But the search for legal, safe, effective performance improvement never ends. In the last thirty or forty years, many (if not most) elite athletes, at the peak of their health and fitness, seeking to improve performance even further, have resorted to: Chiropractic. Chiropractic is natural, works with the body, safe (low malpractice rates), effective, and most important: legal performance improvement.

Chiropractic improves the body mind connection (the nervous system). Chiropractic removes interference along the lines of communication (the nerves). Chiropractic is preventative for injury because Chiropractic improves proprioception (back to the "body-mind" connection but with a technical term). Chiropractic is wonderful for rehabilitation post-injury; restoring proper alignment, motion, and again, that proprioception connection.

When our healthiest, fittest, strongest, fastest, disease free, injury free, demographic seeks out Chiropractic care to optimize their physiology, structure, neurology, does it not evidence that that Chiropractic is indeed: "Beyond the Back"? Most of us are NOT elite athletes, but when the *best* athletes in their prime seek Chiropractic care, does it not make sense that Chiropractic would benefit any and all of us? Whether we are a senior looking to prevent a fall (balance, proprioception); a weekend warrior looking to prevent injury; the average person looking to return from injury; or a person with almost any health condition - Chiropractic will benefit you!

Why is Chiropractic 'Beyond The Back'?

"Beyond the Back", yes- a great title; a regimen of Chiropractic is far reaching. Chiropractic does indeed have good effects well 'beyond the back'. Due to nervous system connections, Chiropractic can reach every fiber of your being, and help it heal!

What's the History of Chiropractic Care For Athletes?

Almost one hundred years ago, this 'performance improvement effect' was already known. The greatest athletes were already using Chiropractic - the New York Yankees! The following is taken from a newspaper (The Denver Post - Sunday Morning, October 14, 1928; Section One, Page Nine) - an actual page from the newspaper that I have hanging on my office wall - (direct quotes from this contemporaneous article are italicized):

"..... Health for the New York Yankees meant the World's Championship AND a large financial gain; likewise, health means success for you in your endeavor. Without health, you can only be an "also ran".

Chiropractic maintained the health of the Yanks and they succeeded throughout the most grueling season of their history. Chiropractic has a similar value for EVERY individual.

Dr. Al Woods, D.C., trainer of the Yanks, (throughout the entire Yank Managing career of Miller Huggins), was voted a PLAYER'S FULL SHARE of the World Series Grand Prize. Dr. Woods did not carry a bat nor throw a ball. The Yankee players voted him an EQUAL share with them in appreciation of the value of his Chiropractic Services..." [1]

If you enjoy sports, if you enjoy Major League Baseball, you know of the NY Yankee Dynasty (ultimately with 27 World Series championships and 40 American League pennants) in 1921, the Yankees made their first World Series Appearance. In the years since their first appearance, the Yankees have been in the 'Big Game' almost 40% of the time. In the 95 years since their first appearance, the Yankees have won 27 out of 40 appearances or 68% of the time. They were cared for by Dr. Al Woods, DC, then followed by Dr. Erle V Painter, DC, who was there throughout the 1930's. The NY Yankees, an elite team, knew of the value of Chiropractic towards improving performance.

The NY Yankees employed Chiropractors as their trainers before Chiropractic was licensed in New York State, and tried to keep this performance improvement, health giving, approach their own secret.

Baseball fans debate 'who is the best team of all time'? Often the answer is the 1927 Yankees. In the 1920's, the NY Yankees Head Coach was Miller Huggins ('Hug'). Coach Huggins showed up with the Yankees in 1918 and stayed through 1929. The Yankees were in the World Series in 1921, '22, '23, '26, '27, '28.

Dr. Al Woods, Chiropractor; was with the NY Yankees for that entire run.

Chiropractic helped the Yankee 1927 World Series Championship team to become a legend. Babe Ruth, Lou Gehrig, Bob Meusel, Earle Combs, Tony Lazzeri, Joe Dugan, Bob Shawkey, Herb Pennock, Waite Hoyt, and the whole team performed to their best with Chiropractic at their side.

In the decade of the 1920's, the Yankees established a dynasty. In the 1920's, the Yankees had among the lowest days lost to sickness or injury in the baseball industry. In the decade of the 1920's, the Yankees had a Doctor of Chiropractic as their primary health care provider. Obviously, Dr. Woods, the team trainer referred out when appropriate, but Chiropractic prevented injury and restored health before more invasive or other forms of care were necessary.

In part, this newspaper article shows a picture of the 1928 Yankee team. 28 men are pictured: 25 players, one coach (Miller Huggins), a mascot (bat boy), and a "trainer," Dr. Al Woods, Doctor of Chiropractic.

The article includes a picture of a Western Union telegram of the era confirming that Dr. Woods was indeed a graduate of the Carver Chiropractic Institute.[2] Dr. Al Woods, trainer of the best team ever, was a Doctor of Chiropractic - forty years before Chiropractic was licensed in the state of New York![3]

If Chiropractic helped Babe Ruth and Lou Gherig, do you think it could help you? If Chiropractic is helping Professional and Olympic athletes break records today, do you think it could help you? If Chiropractic leads to fewer sick days (60% less hospital admissions, 59% less days in the hospital, 62% less outpatient surgeries, 85% less in pharmaceutical costs)[4] do you think that could help you? If chiropractic led to fewer injuries[5] do you think it could help you? If you run a company, employ people, do you want fewer sick days, fewer injuries, better productivity (improved performance)? Then you want a regimen of Chiropractic! If you have a family, do you want fewer sick days? Then you want preventive care at your local Doctor of Chiropractic! If you work for yourself; and absolutely, positively HAVE to show up and be there at work-- then you want a regular schedule of Chiropractic evaluation and adjustment!

One of the sports and fitness gurus from the 20th century who continued into our 21st century was Dr. Jack LaLanne, DC. Jack was a television fitness instructor from the 1950s through the time of his death. Whether on his own show or as a guest; whether as a competitor or ultimately a television health celebrity, Jack was an example of what the Chiropractic lifestyle could bring each and every one of us: a healthy, fit, active life well into our nineties!

Examples exist from history through today of increased health, and performance improvement enjoyed by our fittest athletes through Chiropractic care. The 'general population' should take notice and improve their health through the same safe, natural, noninvasive, effective way the above legends did- by utilizing Chiropractic.

What are some of the concepts for Sports Chiropractioc?

There are a few important concepts for 'Sports' Chiropractic: Efficiency, habituation, nociception, facilitation, mechanoreceptors, biomechanics, body/mind connection, adaptation, neuroplasticity, subluxation, and adjustment.

Habituation is when the body adapts and establishes patterns in our brain and body. Posture and repetitive movements become a pattern in the body, which become habits. We can build efficient, stress free adaptive patterns that build health, or inefficient stressful patterns that build or predispose us to injury or disease. Posture is an example, a product of habituation. Dr Thomas Harris, a medical doctor, is quoted as saying; "Changes in the optimal spinal position produce spinal pathologies and loss of function. Spinal pathologies destroy joint reflexes, arc fibers and cause nerve impedance. Postural strength and coordination are essential for injury prevention and sports performance."[6]

In the quote above, it appears that this MD could be describing a spinal subluxation, which is exactly what chiropractors seek and treat. **Subluxation** has been discussed at many a conference and in academic circles. Of note: Chung Ha Suh, PhD (Spinal Biomechanics Expert, University of Colorado) is quoted as saying, "Subluxation is very real. We have documented it to the extent that no one can dispute its existence. Vertebral Subluxations change the entire health of the body by causing structural dysfunction of the spine and nerve interference. The weight of a dime on a spinal nerve will reduce nerve transmission by as much as sixty percent."

A subluxation does not have to cause pain. But a misalignment or motion dysfunction is going to set up what is called nociception in the spine. **Nociception** is the sensory nervous system's response to harmful or potentially harmful stimuli. Nociception may or may not hit the threshold of the conscious perception of pain. Pain may take time and summation to develop. Pain is felt *after* the dysfunction or damage has been done!

Nociception is where the nervous system starts to talk to the brain and says 'something is wrong here'. When it starts to say that, it is creating static, creating stress in the system, so that the brain cannot listen to other messages. Nociception is the body talking to the brain - enough nociception and the brain cannot be as efficient handling other incoming messages.

The brain accepts messages from the body. The brain also sends messages to the body. When stress (nociception) is in the system, along the pathway; when the brain sends a message down the spinal cord to an arm, a leg, a heart, a lung, or a stomach, that transmission is altered. When you have a dysfunctioning nerve, you're going to have a dysfunctioning cell at the end of that nerve. If things are dysfunctioning for an athlete, you are not going to have your best performance. Athletes want optimal performance; 'Joe Average' may just want improved health.

Sports Chiropractic is a non-invasive, safe, effective and cost-effective approach towards improving performance and health. Sports Chiropractic is preventive of injury by finding and correcting stress and interference in the communications system of the body. The brain communicates with the cells, tissues, muscles and organs in the body through the spinal cord and nerves. Chiropractic improves that communication, hence improves performance and lessens risk of injury.

When there is a biomechanical stress (i.e.: vertebral subluxation), that stress alters the transmission along the nerves, which alters input and output of the nervous system. Once the biomechanical fault creates that neurological alteration, there are physiologic consequences that can result in ineffective muscle firing, imbalance, injury and illness within that body. The Chiropractor evaluates and treats for that biomechanical stress, corrects that stress (subluxation) through a Chiropractic adjustment, relieves the neurological alteration, and restores homeostatic physiologic function. That is preventive, performance improving, Sports Chiropractic.

Gray's Anatomy states that every organ, system and function of the human body is under direct control of the central nervous system.[7]

How long have you been a Sports Chiropractor?

I've been in practice for almost 35 years, and I have all kinds of patients. I have a general Chiropractic practice but my interests lay in sports injuries and sports Chiropractic. I enjoy sports – although I was never good at them – and I've always been a fan. "Sports" Chiropractic is a Doctor of Chiropractic at the field, court, or event. Once the patient enters the Chiropractic office, the difference is minimal between a "Sports" Chiropractor and a "regular" Chiropractor. Most Chiropractors utilize a wide array of modalities in the office setting, but the key approach is to seek the subluxation and correct the subluxation with adjustment if found.

Chiropractic helps all kinds of people – from infants to people in their nineties, athletes and non-athletes. Of course, I take care of people with injuries sustained from automobile accidents or workplace injuries. My office cares for just about any type of neuro-muscular-skeletal type of injury or complaint, strains and sprains, and those general complaints that many people have which are also applicable to athletes and sports injuries. It is much more common to get a bruise, a strain, a sprain in sports than it is to actually fracture something or cause a dislocation (off to the Orthopedic MD for those!).

Chiropractic is very applicable to the athlete or the general patient. The general public can hurt themselves just stepping off a curb, lifting something heavy, sitting too long at work, or sleeping improperly. An athlete can injure themselves from overuse, overtraining, doing too much too soon, or some type of actual traumatic injury such as when a football player gets hit and gets a strain, sprain, or bruise.

Chiropractic is applicable across a broad range of conditions. Often, even today, some patients show up for common complaints of headache, neck stiffness, back pain, sciatica or a disc problem. These conditions respond to Chiropractic, but patients frequently find that other symptoms or complaints respond as well! Some of my patients have said to me that 'Chiropractic is far reaching'; hence the title of our book "Beyond the Back".

If it's not a fracture or dislocation (which is relatively rare and would be referred to the orthopedic surgeon), the Chiropractic office is a good place for the general public or an athlete to come, initiate care, have an examination/ evaluation/ and perhaps treatment or referral to another discipline.

Why did you choose to be a Chiropractor?

My whole family went to chiropractors, including my great-grandparents who lived well in to their nineties. Even in their eighties and nineties, my grandparents used to crawl into the Chiropractic clinic and then dance their way out. My family is particularly long lived, living into their nineties routinely, and with vitality. I think part of the reason is that my family has always gone to the chiropractor.

I'm the first chiropractor in the family and I do take care of my entire family. Given risk factors, and given expectations in my family, my family generally uses no medication or uses less medication than our contemporaries. We are also generally more active than our contemporaries and I think certainly a whole lot of that good health is due to receiving regular Chiropractic care. Becoming a Doctor of Chiropractic was a natural for me. I love helping people naturally, safely, effectively. I enjoy helping people after other approaches have failed to ameliorate their complaint(s).

My primary interest is sports injuries. I have a credential in sports injuries, called the DACBSP, Diplomate of the American Chiropractic

Board of Sports Physicians. I have an International Certified Chiropractic Sports Practitioner (ICSSP), awarded by the International Federation of Sports Chiropractic/Fédération Internationale de Chiropratique du Sport (FICS). I have an Emergency Medical Technician Certification (EMT); I've ridden an ambulance in the 911 emergency system of New York City. I've also taught classes in nursing school, and recently became a registered nurse (RN) myself. Of course, I have my Doctor of Chiropractic license. I have a broad and unique background in several levels of healthcare and across professional disciplines. All of this helps me on the sidelines where I may be the only health professional, or I may be part of a team of health professionals with medical doctors, physical therapists, athletic trainers, massage therapists, even nutritionists, acupuncturists, and all types of disciplines. Sports Chiropractors can function ALONE or as part of a multi-disciplinary team of health professionals.

Why Chiropractic for Athletes?

Whether you are an athlete, or "just a regular person", there's that saying again: "Chiropractic adds life to your years and years to your life." I think you can translate that into the sports world as well. Chiropractic does increase performance because it makes the body a more efficient machine. A more efficient machine means fewer symptoms, fewer injuries, and a longer healthier career. For 'Joe or Joan Olympic' or 'Joe or Joan Professional Athlete', it makes them function better and that creates performance improvement through the natural working of the body. Working with Mother Nature, Chiropractic is probably much more heavily utilized in the elite sports world than in the "average" American world. The vast majority of professional, Olympic, and elite athletes make Chiropractic care part of their sports health team, while most Americans use Chiropractic almost solely for pain, and do not normally, routinely use chiropractors to improve their health.

The sports health team, the 'medical' staff for athletes, could include medical doctors, orthopedists, dentists, psychiatrists, physical therapists, massage therapists, nutritionists, acupuncturists, as well as the chiropractor. Each of these disciplines and professions has their own focus. Certainly all of them may work on sprains and strains. For example, the psychiatrist might work on a 'sprained' athlete's mood, emotions, cognition, and their state of mind. If an athlete gets hurt, certainly a physical therapist or a massage therapist is going to work on a sprain or strain and make sure the muscles, ligaments, the soft tissue, and the hard tissue maintains its integrity. The chiropractor looks at all of this and, in particular, looks at alignment of the spine, the alignment of any/all joints. Each discipline has its own specialty, and its own concerns and approach.

Chiropractors are neuro-bio-mechanical experts. Analysis of gait, motion, and posture can help an athlete or a non-athlete prevent injuries, or rehabilitate from a trauma, or an injury. Often, at an elite level, chiropractors are part of a larger health staff, but sometimes when we work at the college, high school, or 'pee-wee' level-- we may be the only medical professional on site. So sometimes the chiropractor may massage, may tape, or may even act similarly to a sports psychologist to help the athlete over their psychological-mental fear and upset over an injury or over an impending long rehabilitation period.

I've been at games where I have been the ONLY health professional— as have my sports chiropractor colleagues—and sometimes a competitor goes down with a severe injury, spinal injury, dislocation, concussion, or even possibly a heart attack—a very emergent condition. Often the sports chiropractor, outside of the higher level sports, functions almost as a 'jack of all trades', almost functioning as multiple disciplines.

Can you give an example where Sports Chiropractic helped an athlete?

Myself and a couple of other chiropractors were functioning as the primary health providers at a Professional Rodeo several years ago. We were all certified sports Chiropractic physicians. At this event, an athlete got bucked off a horse. Horses are different than bulls – usually when you get bucked off a horse, the horse is happy and he runs away. When you get bucked off a bull, the bull is usually mean and mad and he wants to hurt you. The bull will step on you or butt you or gore you with his horns. Well, this guy was bucked off a horse, and inadvertently, as the cowboy lay on the ground, the horse stepped on his lower right chest/upper right abdomen. Then the horse happily galloped away.

The athlete got up and started walking towards the sidelines, but then suddenly collapsed. Well, when you see somebody get up, walk, and then collapse, it's not a good sign. It shows things are hemodynamically changing. Something bad is going on when someone is initially 'okay', and then there is a change, and suddenly they are 'not okay'. So you have to figure out what that change is, what is going on in that body to cause the collapse.

We entered the arena, took the shirt off the cowboy, and he was actually wearing a flak vest. He had expected to be thrown, so he was looking for self-preservation. We cut off his shirt, then we cut off his flak vest, which was tied in place. In spite of the flak vest, a hoof print over his upper right abdominal quadrant or lower right chest was clearly visible. I knew immediately that he had abdominal injuries, probably a lacerated liver and was probably bleeding inside.

There was an ambulance on scene, assisting with care at the Rodeo. The Chiropractors and Emergency Medical Technicians (EMTs) worked as a team. We placed the patient on an immobilization spine board for fear of a possible spinal injury that could be concurrent with the abdominal bleed. The cowboy was placed into MAST pants (Military anti-shock trousers, or pneumatic anti-shock garments (PASG). These are medical devices used to treat severe blood loss. This was protocol at the time of this injury; and now it is no longer current protocol. Changes in protocol are an example why the sports chiropractor must keep current with changes in standards of care. The ambulance gave advance notification, quickly transported him to the hospital, and within 20 minutes of leaving the rodeo field, he was having emergency abdominal surgery to repair his lacerated liver and lacerated intestines, which saved his life.

You can't always make that diagnosis quickly, but we were properly trained, and immediately recognized the severity of the injury. Off he went to the hospital, properly packaged with instructions from me, and emergency surgery literally saved his life. Delay in this critical diagnosis or treatment would have cost this cowboy his life, as he would have bled out internally. That same night, a representative came to the Rodeo site and thanked the chiropractors for recognizing the critical injury, initiating proper care, and assisting and instructing the ambulance crew as to the extent of suspected injury.

For another example, I was at the Olympic training center for a rotation. A young man came to me who was a gymnast. He had low back problems that had persisted with him for a couple of years, progressively worsening. This young man presented to me on my first day of rotation, and progressively, over weeks of treatment, he improved. I was lucky enough to provide pure Chiropractic care to him, doing some Cox distractive technique upon his lower back (there are many, many Chiropractic techniques from which the DC can choose). At first, he was disabled, unable to compete, but still hopeful to make the travel team and compete in the Olympics. By the time I left that rotation, he had improved to a full 'return to play', gained a spot on the team, and got his Olympic experience.

Pure chiropractic, applied by me, restored his low back to proper motion, and proper alignment. Of course, he was also getting physical therapy and massage therapy, and he was working out with certified strength and conditioning coaches; he had a team of doctors and health professionals working on him. Multiple approaches and disciplines had been working on this patient over a period of several months to a year. Despite these varied approaches, he had been unable to progress and return to his sport. But appropriate Chiropractic manipulation to his spine, within the space of a few weeks, restored him to 90-95% of his function. He was able to go on and compete at an Olympic level thanks to the intervention of Chiropractic, which was different and distinct from all the other treatments he had received.

Speaking of the United States Olympic training center, as I write this, the head man there is a chiropractor. He manages the Olympic training center clinic at Colorado Springs. His name is Dr. Bill Moreau. He is a Doctor of Chiropractic, he also has a DACBSP, Diplomate of American Chiropractic Board of Sports Physicians. He's the guy that the health staff report to. He's the medical director of the USOC and he takes care of the entire USA Olympic team. That is a chiropractor that is running the show at the US OTC, helping our athletes prevent injury, improve performance, and also recover from injury and return to competition.

Have there been studies on athletes?

Yes. A pioneering study tested reaction time of 25 athletes that utilized chiropractic adjustments in their training regimen. This Chiropractic group was compared to 25 athletes with the same training schedule who were not receiving chiropractic adjustments. At six weeks, it was found that the chiropractic group scored significantly better on 11 standard tests of athletic ability (broad jump, vertical jump, side step test, response movement test, hand reaction time, distance perception, etc.).

Impressive changes took place in the chiropractic athletes' reaction times. The control group (non-chiropractic) exhibited less than 1% improvement, while the athletes under chiropractic care achieved reaction times more than 18% faster than their initial scores.[8]

From the American Journal of Pain Management:

> "Posture affects and moderates every physiological function, from breathing to nervous system function. And despite the considerable evidence that posture affects physiology and function, the significant influence of posture on health is not addressed by most physicians."[9]

This quote supports the importance of biomechanics and how those biomechanics can affect the neurology and the physiology of our body. That is what chiropractors look at, the biomechanics of the spine, which houses the central nervous system, which in turn is the control system of the entire body.

J. Edwards, Phd. said in the Journal of Neurological Science (Aug 1994), "The quality of healing is directly proportional to the functional capability of the central nervous system to send and receive nerve messages."[10] After an injury or illness, you are going to heal only as good as your unstressed, subluxation free nervous system directs and allows. The Journal of Neurological Science mirrors what DCs have been saying for decades.

Chiropractic alone looks for that biomechanical dysfunction, looks for that problem termed a subluxation in the spine, which is the home of the nervous system. Then Chiropractic lays hands upon that spine, or shoulder, or elbow, and adjusts that joint and that restores the biomechanical integrity of the joint. Chiropractic care thus also restores the neurological integrity of the nervous system and it allows the body to function better.

Arnold Schwarzenegger won Mr. Olympia seven times. One of his colleagues, Dr. Franco Columbo is a chiropractor. Dr. Columbo said, "The best way to use Chiropractic is not only after injuries, but before the injury occurs." If you think about it, these elite athletes had to prevent injury, therefore had to utilize Chiropractic. Elite body builders work out hours every day, six or seven days a week, every week, month in/month out, year in, year out. That is why they seek Chiropractic care preventatively. Lee Labrada, Mr. Universe, stated, "Chiropractic has helped keep me injury free. That is half the trick to staying in competition."

What is a misconception that people have about sports-related injuries?

A common misconception is that the injuries have to be visible, traumatic, and probably they need surgery. The vast majority of sports injuries are minor traumas that add up over time. You don't have to fall down the stairs or have a car crash to have a problem. You do not have to have a hard tackle or get hit by a pitch to have an injury. Most injuries are minor, mild, and may or may not become progressively symptomatic. Perhaps you're exercising too much and you start to build fatigue into your system. If you're practicing incorrectly then eventually you will have problems in your joints and in your body.

What are some of the common warning signs for athletes?

When you are overworking or overtraining, there are common warning signs that someone can look for when they're getting into what's called exhaustion. They start to feel disinterested and irritable. There's a change in their sleep routine, and they complain about a lack or change of sleep and appetite. They may lose weight unexpectedly. Even their skin can look unhealthy. These things are all signs that the body is going past adaptation and into exhaustion. Look for these signs, before injury, pain or illness develops!

What is a misconception that people have about sports-related injuries?

That injury or illness always develops suddenly. Injury/illness *can* develop suddenly, but more often than not, it develops over time. A well accepted, scientific explanation of that gradual, progressive development is the "General Adaptation Syndrome (GAS)."[11]

Back in the 1930's Dr. Hans Selye, MD, PhD, developed this GAS theory. [12]

Dr. Selye was nominated for the Nobel Prize no less than seventeen times.[13]

This GAS theory is important to know in order to understand building/improving performance, building health, or developing injury or illness. Dr. Selye states: "The beginning of the disease process begins with postural distortions."[14]

Dr. Selye is talking about the initiation of stress in the body, and the process of stress causing illness and injury. Another MD spoke about the endpoint of what this un-addressed stress caused to the body: disease and death. "Organs supplied by impinged nerves exhibit pathological changes and the more serious the impingement, the more serious the damage." -Henry Winsor, M.D., 1921.[15]

Before we discuss Dr. Selye and what stressors (i.e.: Subluxation) do in our body, we must also be aware of a couple of other concepts. Predecessors to Dr. Selye include Claude Bernard (who developed the idea of milieu intérieur) and Walter Cannon's "homeostasis". These concepts had to do with the "Balance" within our body.

To keep balance (technically termed homeostasis) the body must be ever constantly changing. This constant changing in biology and physiology is known as adaptation. Adaptation in the body is mediated by cells communicating with each other. In living bodies, living cells communicate primarily, instantaneously, through the nervous system. Any irritation to that nervous system decreases the ability to react instantaneously, appropriately, efficiently.

An irritation or alteration alters our body's functions, physiology, balance (homeostasis). Altered biomechanics (subluxation) create altered nerve transmission. Altered nerve transmission alters the functions of cells, tissues, organs. That is why elite athletes seek Chiropractic: to remove these alterations, these aberrations and optimize nervous system function which in turn allows a more optimal functioning of every cell, tissue, organ in the entire body.

1. ALARM = a stressor = Something's going on and our body subconsciously, automatically (and sometimes possibly consciously) becomes aware of the stressor.

2. RESISTANCE = adaptation = some type of reaction in the cells, tissues or organ within our body. The nervous system and the endocrine systems release hormonal messages which mobilize the body, things can happen distant from the alarm point.

3. EXHAUSTION = breakdown = if the body cannot handle the stressor and adaptation, if the cells, tissues, organs cannot 'live with it', eventually the system breaks down. The body becomes exhausted if the stress increases drastically or if it's maintained too long.

When we are over stressed, we can no longer adapt. When we can no longer adapt, we become exhausted. When we become exhausted, breakdown occurs. Whether an athlete or a regular person, we want to maximize our adaptative capability. To maximize our adaptive capability, we must minimize stress within our system. To maximize our adaptive capability and reduce stress (static) within the body, we must have good brain-body communication. When we have maximized the efficiency of our brain-body communication we prevent progression to exhaustion.

Upon approaching exhaustion and breakdown, often we make a recommendation of P.R.I.C.E. That recommendation would be the same for athletes and non-athletes: **P**rotection, **R**est, **I**ce, **C**ompression, **E**levation. It's very important to rest appropriately when you're participating in sports. That is when you repair and restore. But also, you don't want to rest too much because prolonged rest leads to deconditioning.

What should athletes do if they are worried they're working too hard?

Something people can do in the quest to prevent injury (besides seeing the chiropractor), is to look at their pulse rate and be aware of changes. If the pulse goes up 10 or more from their normal resting pulse, an injury can result within the next few training days. If the pulse resting rate is up ten or more points than your normal; perhaps it is time to rest!

If you have unexplained weight loss, a sudden drop of three or four percent from a person's normal resting weight, this can be a signal of overwork/overtraining; maybe it is time to rest. The sleep routine, if it's irregular, if it's interrupted, if someone gets 10% less sleep (less than their established normal), that is also a sign they are working too hard or exceeding their adaptive capacity. An inability to achieve your goals, or an inability to finish your last workout indicates the body is being overwhelmed and it may be time for a rest period.

Micro trauma and repetitive stress over time can also lead up to a significant injury. I often ask people, "What is stronger, a drip of water or a boulder?" Well, over time, a drip of water will wear a hole through that boulder. The Grand Canyon was cut by a river. It's the same with us. Over time, if we are biomechanically misaligned, we're going to put too much stress on our joints and over time we will get an injury.

This is the Chiropractic forte, looking for the biomechanical lesion, the subluxation, which leads to dysfunction in that joint, and can lead to joint, connective tissue problems. Again, think of the cascade of effects related to the biomechanical dysfunction; ultimately that stress in the system leads to neurological and physiological consequences.

The chiropractor can help a person heal before (prevention) and after injury (restoration, recuperation, rehabilitation). Increased performance coincides with an increased health and fitness.

"Postural strength and coordination are essential for injury prevention and sports performance"

Thomas Harris, MD, The Sports Medicine Guide

A few words on Concussion

As this chapter is written, Concussion is a major topic amongst sports medicine specialists. I have been on the sidelines, on the mat, on the field, and on the court for over thirty years at sporting events. Rodeo, Football, Tae Kwon Do, Judo, Karate, Basketball, Rugby, Soccer, even Professional Bowling are some of the events that I have covered. With this background, I have seen more than a few concussions at events, and also later on in the office.

Of note: a concussion will usually also involve the vertebral subluxation complex. It can take 90 G's of force to cause a concussion, although concussion can also occur due to much lower forces.[16] It takes less than

10 G's of force to cause a 'whiplash' (cervical acceleration/deceleration injury CAD). If you have a concussion, you are probably going to have a degree of whiplash. With that concussion, you likely have a CAD and the associated cervical misalignment/motion aberration (subluxation).

With that cervical spine/cervical neurology altered, you are going to have your autonomic nervous system function altered. That means the blood vessel tone is altered in your brain. In the aftercare of concussion, you may want to get your cervical spine checked for a subluxation, which was inevitably caused if you have a concussion. You want to reduce that subluxation so that your blood vessels function properly. When you feed your brain the right amount of blood and oxygen, the brain and body can heal itself better. Based upon this autonomic nervous system involvement, Chiropractic should be part of the aftercare in the diagnosis of 'concussion'.

When the brain and body are not well connected; for example, when an athlete has a concussion, if they return to play too soon, they are almost four times more likely to have an ACL tear.[17]

What does a knee have to do with a concussion? It seems pretty distant. The relationship is indirect. But the relationship is there. The relationship exists because the concussion in the brain alters the way the brain functions. The relationship exists because the concussion has an alteration in the brain and concomitant alteration in the neurology of the cervical spine. Perhaps the brain has recovered, but if the cervical spine is not checked, the message between the brain and body is still distorted, and the reaction time is slower, muscles fire incorrectly to stabilize that knee. If the nerves are altered and the muscles are not firing properly, the possibility of injury increases.

This is where Chiropractic is different from massage therapy, or physical therapy, or the orthopedist, who gives medication or performs surgery. We work structurally, but be aware that structure affects the neurology, which affects the physiology. I am not saying that Chiropractic is the answer to concussion (or any/every health problem), however, I am saying that Chiropractic should be part of the multi-disciplinary health team that evaluates and perhaps treats (as needed) a concussion patient.

Conclusion

Sports Chiropractic:

- Has been utilized in the elite sports world for over a hundred years (i.e.: NY Yankee Championship teams)

- Has a long track record of success

- Benefits structural (biomechanical) problems

- Removes stress/static/irritation from the nervous system

- Restores/maintains balance and homeostasis

- Prevents problems

- Improves performance

- 'Adds life to years and years to life'

- Affects all of these biological, neurological, physiological functions

If the world's best athletes, a super healthy population, seek out Chiropractic care to improve the functioning of their machine (their body) don't you think the 'average' person would benefit from a Chiropractic evaluation and treatment regimen?

Citations:

1. THE DENVER POST-- "The Best Newspaper in the U. S. A."--Sunday Morning, October 14, 1928; Section One, Page Nine

2. THE DENVER POST-- "The Best Newspaper in the U. S. A."--Sunday Morning, October 14, 1928; Section One, Page Nine

3. NYS Chiropractic Licensure; https://www.nysca.com/history.asp ; http://www.nysca.com/w/newsphotos/S3345.jpg

4. Journal of Manipulative and Physiological Therapy, MAY 2007; 30(4): 263-269, Richard L. Samat, MD, James Winterstein, DC, Jerrilyn A. Cambron, DC, PhD

5. BMC Musculoskeletal Disorders201011:64 , DOI: 10.1186/1471-2474-11-64, © Hoskins and Pollard; licensee BioMed Central Ltd. 2010 ; The effect of a sports chiropractic manual therapy intervention on the prevention of back pain, hamstring and lower limb injuries in semi-elite Australian Rules footballers: a randomized controlled trial

6. Harris, Thomas; The Sports Medicine Guide For the Everyday Athlete, Slawson Communications (October 1989)

7. Gray, H.; Grays Anatomy (1987) Bounty Books

8. Lauro A, Mouch B. Chiropractic effects on athletic ability. J Chiropractic Research and Clinical Investigation, 1991; 6:84-87.)

9. Lennon, J. (1994, Jan.) American Journal of Pain Management

10. Edwards, J. (1994, August) "Nerve dysfunction and tissue healing." Journal of Neurological Science

11. http://medical-dictionary.thefreedictionary.com/ general+adaptation+syndrome, http://www.currentnursing.com/nursing_theory/Selye's_stress_theory.html

12. Hans Selye; Nature (1936, 138(3479):32)

13. http://www.nobelprize.org/nomination/archive/show_people.php?id=8395

14. Seyle, Hans; The Stress of Life, (1978) McGraw-Hill Publishing

15. Windsor Autopsies; https://vimeo.com/108909014; Sympathetic Segmental Disturbances- 11. The Evidence of the Association, in Dissected Cadavers, of Visceral Disease with Vertebral Deformities of the Same Sympathetic Segments, The Medical Times, Nov. 1921, pps, 267- 271 ; Windsor Autopsies; http://www.dorn-method.com /pdf/WinsorMDArticleSympatheticSegmentalDisturbances.pdf

16. UCLA Today, Making football helmets safer to prevent concussions, Mike Fricano | August 22, 2013

17. Herman D, Jones D, Harrison A, et al. Concussion increases the risk of subsequent lower extremity musculoskeletal injury in collegiate athletes. Clin J Sport Med. 2013;23:124.

About the Author

Dr Victor Dolan

121 Parkinson Ave
Staten Island, NY
Phone: 718-981-9755
Website: www.drvictordolan.net

Dr. Dolan also answers questions at
www.allexperts.com/el/Chiropractors

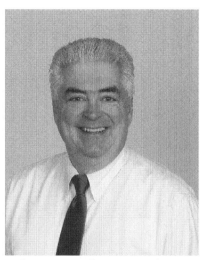

Dr. Victor E. Dolan, Doctor of Chiropractic; was the first Chief of Chiropractic in any Hospital in New York State (DHSI). This extraordinary feat was recognized by the Governor of New York State, the NYS State Senate, NYS Assembly; and the New York City Council. Dr. Dolan received national recognition from Prevention Magazine for integrating Chiropractic into the Hospital setting. He has been invited to care for USA Olympic Athletes at the US Olympic Training Center. Dr. Dolan has been selected to the Medical Staff of the Pan American Games, the Caribbean American Games, and the World Sport Games. Dr. Dolan is Team Chiropractor to the Championship NYPD Football Team, the PSAL Curtis High School Football team (for 30 years) and has been named to the Staten Island SPORTS Hall of Fame as an Unsung Hero. Dr. Dolan is also an Emergency Medical Technician and a licensed Registered Nurse.

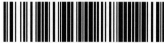

Made in the USA
Charleston, SC
10 March 2017